Teaching Nursing

NURSING PROGRAM
NEUMANN COLLEGE
ASTON, PA. 19014

Teaching Nursing

Sandra DeYoung, EdD

The William Paterson College of New Jersey

Addison-Wesley Nursing
A Division of The Benjamin/Cummings Publishing Company, Inc.

Redwood City, California • Fort Collins, Colorado • Menlo Park, California
Reading, Massachusetts • New York • Don Mills, Ontario • Wokingham, U.K.
Amsterdam • Bonn • Sydney • Singapore • Tokyo • Madrid • San Juan

Sponsoring Editor: Debra Hunter
Production Coordinator: John Walker
Copy Editor: Jackie Estrada
Text Design and Composition: Merry Finley, Desktop Productions
Cover Design: Betty Gee, Side by Side Studios

Library of Congress Cataloging-in-Publication Data

DeYoung, Sandra.
    Teaching nursing / Sandra DeYoung.
      p.   cm.
    ISBN 0-201-09265-4
      1. Nursing—Study and teaching. I. Title.
      [DNLM: 1. Education, Nursing. 2. Teaching—methods. WY 18
    D529t]
    RT71.D55   1989
    610.73'07—dc20
    DNLM/DLC
    for Library of Congress   89-17805
                                                CIP

ISBN 0-201-09265-4

ABCDEFGHIJK-BA-892109

Addison-Wesley Nursing
A Division of The Benjamin/Cummings Publishing Company, Inc.
390 Bridge Parkway
Redwood City, CA 94065

Dedicated to my family and friends,
who encourage and support all my efforts.

Preface

Many nurses in graduate schools today will find that formal teaching is a part of their work role even if they are not full-time teachers. Therefore, many graduate students benefit from taking at least one course in the theory and methods of nursing education.

This text is designed to introduce graduate students to the basics of education—how students (whether they are generic nursing students or RNs) learn, and how teachers can best help them to learn. It is a compilation of information from research, from my own experience as an educator for the past seventeen years, and from great minds in the field of education.

Too often new teachers teach as they were taught, using the same methods over and over, not even sure why these methods are used. Teaching should be much more scientific than that; we cannot rest on tradition but must apply what research has taught us about learning and effective teaching. We have to make the best use of the limited time that we have with students to teach them not just facts but how to learn and how to solve problems.

Instructors already in the classroom who have not had courses in education could also benefit from studying this book. All of us, whether we have been in teaching for two months or twenty years, can improve our teaching. We must all be continuous learners.

Chapter 1 is a summary of research on what makes a "good" teacher, especially in the eyes of the students; this is a topic everyone should find interesting. Chapter 2 is a summary of learning theory that is important to nursing education. The information in this chapter provides a basis for all the methodology to follow. Chapter 3 contains practical advice for how to go about planning and conducting classes, from writing objectives through writing test questions. The remaining eight chapters deal with teaching methods or techniques that can be applied in the classroom, college nursing laboratory, or clinical setting.

The teacher of a generic course in nursing education or an in-service educator can use this text as a basis for lectures, discussions, role playing, seminars, and so on, that will help apply, illustrate, and bring to life the theory being taught.

Sandra DeYoung

Reviewers

Kathleen G. Burke, CCRN, MSN
Instructor, Critical Care Track,
  Graduate Program
School of Nursing
University of Pennsylvania

Kathleen B. Gaberson, RN, PhD
Assistant Professor, Graduate
  Program
School of Nursing
Duquesne University

Carol Gilbert, RN, PhD
Chairperson, Full Professor
Department of Nursing
Fitchburg State College

Sybil M. Lassiter, RN, PhD
Associate Professor
School of Nursing
Adelphi University

Deitra L. Lowdermilk, RNC, PhD
Clinical Associate Professor
School of Nursing
The University of North Carolina at
  Chapel Hill

Patricia Lynch, RN, EdD
Director of Education and
  Training
Sequoia Hospital
Redwood City, California

Helen S. O'Shea, RN, PhD
Professor
Nell Hodgson Woodruff School
  of Nursing
Emory University

Roberta Olson, RN, PHD
Associate Professor
School of Nursing
University of Kansas

Sharon Braund Reed, RN, PHN,
  BSN
Home Health Nurse
San Diego, California

Jo Stejskal, RN, MSN
Associate Professor, Department
  of Nursing
College of Nursing and Health
  Sciences
Winona State University

Contents

PART

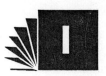

TEACHING
AND LEARNING

Chapter 1

The Good Teacher

Students can easily identify their "good" teachers and "bad" teachers, and they may even be able to distinguish some of the qualities that determine whether teachers are "good" or "bad." Yet, when these students become teachers themselves, they may not find it so easy to follow in the footsteps of their good role models. Different skills are required for subjectively evaluating a teacher than for *being* a good teacher, just as different skills are needed to be a theater critic than to be a good actor.

The effective teacher does not become so just by imitating former good teachers. The process also involves a knowledge of educational theory and research; a willingness to learn new roles, new styles of interacting, and new teaching methods; and the ability to critique one's own performance. Some people have inherent qualities that increase the likelihood of their being good teachers, and they can improve on their natural abilities to make themselves excellent teachers. Those less well endowed with natural talent can still become good teachers, given the proper education, support, and desire to succeed. If it were not possible for "bad" teachers to become better teachers and "good" teachers to become even better than they are by nature, education courses and texts such as this would be a waste of time.

Effective Teaching Behaviors

Considerable research has been devoted to the question of what makes a good teacher. Most of the studies have surveyed students to determine their opinions—a logical method of asking the consumer to evaluate the quality of a product. Student surveys have inherent weaknesses, however. Although the majority of students in a class may agree on the qualities of a good teacher, some students will have differing opinions based on their individual learning styles, goals, and personal needs. It has been found, too, that students tend to emphasize personal or social aspects of teaching behaviors rather than intellectual characteristics (Yamamoto & Dizney, 1966). Conversely, administrators and colleagues often emphasize such qualities as creativity because they have different goals in mind, such as contributions to the college or profession (Tennyson, Boutwell & Frey, 1978). Wotruba and Wright (1975) asked administrators, faculty, and students to rank the importance of ten teacher behaviors in determining teacher effectiveness. Administrators ranked "motivates students to do their best work" as most important, whereas faculty said the most important quality was to be "concerned about fair evaluation of students." Students ranked "evidences a broad, accurate, up-to-date knowledge of the subject" as number one.

Despite the weaknesses of survey methods, such research has provided some useful insights into the components of good teaching. Following is a discussion of behaviors that students and faculty generally agree contribute to effective teaching, even though these groups may rank some of the behaviors differently.

Interpersonal Relationships with Students

An effective teacher is skillful in interpersonal relationships. This skill is demonstrated in taking a personal interest in students, being sensitive to students' feelings and problems, conveying respect for students, alleviating students' anxieties, being accessible for conferences, being fair in all dealings with others, permitting students to express differing points of view, creating an atmosphere in which students feel free to ask questions, and conveying a sense of warmth (Armington et al, 1972; Barham, 1965; Brewer & Brewer, 1970; Brown, 1981; Jacobson, 1966; Kiker, 1973; Lowery et al, 1971; O'Shea & Parsons, 1979; Wong, 1978).

Many teachers with well-developed interpersonal skills find that good relationships with students evolve almost automatically. Others have to become aware of their deficiencies and work on improvement. Viewing students as worthwhile individuals who have something to offer the nursing profession helps keep relationships with them in perspective. It is also helpful to remember the old adage, "Today's student is tomorrow's colleague."

Unfortunately, some teachers believe that showing concern for and interest in students leads to lack of discipline in the classroom, with students taking advantage of their relationship with the teacher. There is no evidence that this belief is accurate; in fact, there is considerable evidence that good student-teacher relationships enhance learning. Carl Rogers (1969) summarized a collection of studies indicating that students actually learn more in classrooms where teachers are student oriented and empathic.

Rogers identified several components of positive interpersonal relationships that he considered applicable to all human interactions, including those in the classroom. These components are *empathy*, or understanding the world as the student sees it; *congruence*, or genuineness in interactions with students; and *positive regard*, or respect for students. Interestingly, as Karns and Schwab (1982) point out, Rogers's concepts are often used and taught by nurse educators in relation to therapeutic communication with patients. These concepts need only be put into practice by teachers whose objective is to establish a trusting relationship with students in order to guide them toward their educational goals.

Nursing students are often plagued by lack of self-confidence and by fear of making mistakes in the clinical area, which leads them to experience high levels of stress. While some anxiety contributes to learning, too much anxiety interferes with the ability to learn. Nursing faculty can help students maintain self-esteem and minimize anxieties by using three basic therapeutic approaches: empathic listening, acceptance, and honest communication.

As in all relationships, it is important that teachers listen to students and try to see the world through their eyes. This approach requires faculty to respect students and care about their concerns and try to understand the world as students experience it.

The second approach is to accept students as they are, whether or not one likes them. Affirming the fact that students are worthwhile people, even though they may be different from oneself, enhances their self-esteem and convinces them that one has faith in their desire and ability to learn. This faith is often rewarded by the students' attempts to live up to the teacher's expectations.

Honest communication is the third ingredient contributing to healthy relationships with students. Students need to know something about the teacher's thoughts regarding the profession of nursing and regarding the students' abilities and performance. If students are not meeting a teacher's expectations, they should know it as soon as possible. No learner should progress through an entire clinical rotation or inservice orientation, for example, to be told only at the end that he or she is not doing well. On the other hand, learners who are doing a superb job should be told so; it is not necessary to search for weaknesses to write on an evaluation if they don't exist.

It is disconcerting for students to be in the dark about what the teacher is thinking. Openness between teacher and students creates a relaxed atmosphere in which students are able to see the teacher as a role model. Students are also better able to handle and accept criticism of their work if the teacher has established an honest and caring relationship with them.

Another aspect of honest communication is clearly identifying the students' responsibilities in the learning process. If students know exactly what is expected of them and what they have to do to succeed, their anxieties will be lessened and the teacher's frustrations will be minimized.

These basic necessities for establishing good relationships with students are not unique to education or to nursing—they are the same components needed for all interpersonal relationships. If students experience them in the teacher-student relationship, they may learn how to incorporate them into other relationships, especially with their patients.

It is easy to understand why students often rate the interpersonal and social aspects of teaching as most important in the learning process. They realize that they are more comfortable with and learn better from teachers who have good interpersonal skills.

Professional Competence

The second hallmark of the good teacher is professional competence. Students and colleagues value a teacher who has a thorough knowledge of the subject matter and can present material in an interesting, clear, and organized manner. The teacher who displays confidence in his or her professional abilities, is creative and stimulating, can excite student interest in the subject, and can demonstrate skills with expertise is rated high (Armington et al, 1972; Brewer & Brewer, 1970; Brown, 1981; Dixon & Koerner, 1976; Gadzella, 1968; Jacobson, 1966; Kiker, 1973; Lowery et al, 1971; Tennyson et al, 1978).

Professional competence has several aspects. The teacher who aims at excellence develops a thorough knowledge of subject matter and polishes skills not only in school but throughout his or her career. He or she maintains and expands this knowledge through reading, research, clinical practice, and continuing education. The competent teacher also learns from life experiences and from students and incorporates all of this knowledge into classroom teaching.

Presenting the subject matter to students in an organized, clear, and interesting manner is a skill that can be learned. This topic is addressed in Chapter 3, but it deserves a few words here. Organization of subject matter requires careful planning to ensure that material is presented logically. Clarity is a variable that is not necessarily planned for but that becomes part of a teacher's style. Researchers have found that the clear teacher is one who uses simple terms to present new material, constantly assesses whether students are understanding and can follow the teacher's train of thought, uses examples whenever possible, allows students time to think about what is being taught, and uses repetition and summarization periodically. (Kennedy et al, 1978; Land & Smith, 1979). Students appreciate clarity. Teaching subject matter in a stimulating way and inspiring student interest hinge on several factors, including the teacher's style, personality, personal interest in the subject, and use of a variety of teaching strategies. We have all been subject to teachers who, while brilliant, organized, and even clear, lack the ability to present the class material in anything but a boring manner. The content of this book is geared toward helping teachers become more interesting as well as more effective.

Personal Qualities

A good teacher is also characterized by certain personal qualities. Teacher qualities valued by students include enthusiasm, willingness to admit to errors, cheerfulness, consideration, honesty, calmness and poise, a sense of humor, control of anger, flexibility, lack of annoying mannerisms, patience, and a neat appearance (Armington et al, 1972; Bridges et al, 1971; Dixon & Koerner, 1976; Jacobson, 1966; Kiker, 1973; Lowery et al, 1971; O'Shea & Parsons, 1979).

Are there any paragons in the field of education who can lay claim to all of these qualities? Probably not. Maybe over the course of a day or a week an individual can maintain that level of behavior, but over the long haul everyone crumbles under the pressures of teaching and of life. That doesn't mean that teachers should not aim for these high standards of personal behavior—they should, and they as well as their students will benefit from these efforts.

Behavior in the Clinical Laboratory

Nursing students have identified several additional behaviors desirable in an instructor teaching in the clinical laboratory as opposed to the classroom. These behaviors include being available in the clinical area, providing conference time, being willing to help, answering questions freely, allowing students to recognize and correct errors, giving verbal encouragement, showing interest in patients and their care, conveying confidence in the learner, and supervising without taking over (Brown, 1981; Jacobson, 1966; O'Shea & Parsons, 1979; Wong, 1978).

Nursing students demonstrate a need for self-confidence, security, and positive feedback in the clinical area. Nursing faculty have to be aware of the needs of learners in those clinical areas in which uncertainty, change, and stress affect learning. Although learners do not need to be babied, they do need a great deal of guidance and support during clinical learning.

Teacher Style

The interpersonal, professional, and personal aspects of good teaching are all important. But more is involved in being a good teacher than just the skills, techniques, and attributes mentioned thus far. Effective teaching involves another phenomenon sometimes referred to as *teacher style*. Eble (1980) believes that style in teaching is an outgrowth of the teacher's personality and character, which is undoubtedly true. For a distinctive style to emerge, it must emerge from something, and that something is probably not just the intellect, but the essential personality. It is style that makes a teacher memorable, interesting, and worth listening to. It is style that makes good teachers into inspired teachers.

Style goes beyond having certain skills and behaviors. It goes beyond carrying out handy hints in a teacher's handbook. Style is a blending of certain ways of talking, moving, relating, thinking. It is more than the ability to entertain or a sense of humor, although these qualities may play a part in a teacher's style.

If you think back to the inspiring teachers that you have had (probably very few), you may be able to recognize style as an important part of their effectiveness. One professor who stands out in my memory had a unique style. He would often sit on the front of his desk, tell a story related to the topic for the day, then relate the story to the class material. He had a homespun appearance and down-to-earth manner, and he conveyed warmth and enthusiasm. Yet for all of his folksy style, his scholarliness, intelligence, and sincerity were clearly evident.

I can also remember a high school teacher who could perhaps best be described as a gracious lady. She dressed elegantly, moved smoothly, talked beautifully, and had a wonderful sense of humor, but above all, she set a high standard of excellence in her own life and high educational standards for her students. Again, all of this was communicated to the students along with her good interpersonal skills and professional competence.

You may not be able to label a particular teacher's style, but you can see that it is there. It may manifest itself in a pleasant speaking voice and animated gestures. It may be observable in the teacher's skill at timing—knowing how to adapt speed of delivery to the particular class and knowing when they are ready for new material or ready to stop. Humor is often a part of style. It may involve telling funny stories, pointing out the ridiculous in certain human situations, laughing with the students, or laughing at oneself, even in front of a class. Using a variety of teaching strategies is a part of style. A personal style may include willingness to share stories from one's professional experience to illustrate certain points; it may be the ability to evoke emotion in students. All these aspects of style blend with the personal and professional attributes already discussed to make the teacher what he or she is. If the blend is just right, the teacher will be hard to forget.

Can style be taught? And once established, can it be changed? Tuckman and Yates (1980) found that a teacher's style could be shaped by student feedback, although their sample consisted of student teachers whose beginning style might well have been malleable. But even veteran teachers whose habits are set can modify their teaching style if they see the need to do so.

Perhaps the most effective means of changing your style is to discuss your teaching with a knowledgeable peer or consultant who has seen you in action or who has reviewed videotapes of your classes. Discussion of your style can raise your consciousness about it and help you examine it more objectively. Reading books on teacher style can help if you discuss the contents with someone and consider ideas on how to implement what you have read.

Kenneth Eble (1980) has said that an admirable style develops only after years of teaching. There is some truth in this. Style does develop slowly in response to results (or lack of them) in your classes and in response to student and peer evaluations. But because style is also a function of personality and character, for some teachers an admirable style may develop early and continue to evolve into something even better over the years.

One important fact must be kept in mind when evaluating teaching effectiveness and using student evaluations as feedback for teachers. There is no one style, technique, or skill that is effective for all students and for all teaching situations. Teachers hope that their skill helps most of the students and that their style is pleasing and stimulating for the majority. As classes change and subjects vary, teachers have to be flexible, modifying their techniques and style to best meet the requirements of the situation. For those few students who do not learn well because of a teacher's classroom approach and style, some individualized attention may be necessary.

References

Armington CL, Reinikka EA, Creighton H: Student evaluation—threat or incentive? *Nurs Outlook* 1972; 20:789–792.

Barham VZ: Identifying effective behavior of the nursing instructor through critical incidents. *Nurs Res* 1965; 14:65–69.

Brewer RE, Brewer MB: Relative importance of ten qualities for college teaching determined by pair comparisons. *J Educ Res* 1970; 63:243–246.

Bridges CM et al: Characteristics of best and worst college teachers. *Science Educ* 1971; 55:545–553.

Brown ST: Faculty and student perceptions of effective clinical teachers. *J Nurs Educ* (Sept)1981; 20:4–15.

Dixon JK, Koerner B: Faculty and student perceptions of effective classroom teaching in nursing. *Nurs Res* 1976; 25:300–305.

Eble KE: Teaching styles and faculty behaviors. Pages 1–6 in: *Improving Teaching Styles.* Eble KE (editor). Jossey-Bass, 1980.

Gadzella BM: College students' views and ratings of an ideal professor. *College and University* 1968; 44:89–96.

Jacobson MD: Effective and ineffective behavior of teachers of nursing as determined by their students. *Nurs Res* 1966; 15:218–224.

Karns PJ, Schwab TA: Therapeutic communication and clinical instruction. *Nurs Outlook* 1982; 30:39–43.

Kennedy JJ et al: Additional investigations into the nature of teacher clarity. *J Educ Res* 1978; 72:3–10.

Kiker M: Characteristics of the effective teacher. *Nurs Outlook* 1973; 21:721–723.

Land ML, Smith LR: Effect of a teacher clarity variable on student achievement. *J Educ Res* 1979; 72:196–197.

Lowery BJ, Keane AP, Hyman IA: Nursing students' and faculty opinion on student evaluation of teachers. *Nurs Res* 1971; 20:436–439.

O'Shea HS, Parsons MK: Clinical instruction: effective and ineffective teacher behaviors. *Nurs Outlook* 1979; 27:411–415.

Rogers CR: *Freedom to Learn*. Charles E. Merrill, 1969.

Tennyson RD, Boutwell RC, Frey S: Student preferences for faculty teaching styles. *Improving College and University Teaching* 1978; 26:194–197.

Tuckman BW, Yates D: Evaluating the student feedback strategy for changing teacher style. *J Educ Res* 1980; 74:74–77.

Wong S: Nurse-teacher behaviours in the clinical field: apparent effect on nursing students' learning. *J Adv Nurs* 1978; 3:369–372.

Wotruba TR, Wright PL: How to develop a teacher-rating instrument. *J Higher Educ* 1975; 46:653–662.

Yamamoto K, Dizney HF: Eight professors—a study on college students' preferences among their teachers. *J Educ Psych* 1966; 51:146–150.

Chapter 2

The Learning Process

The good teacher is one who is competent in the craft of teaching—that is, one who knows the basic principles and propositions of learning and can incorporate them into the classroom. It is not enough to be well versed in a subject area or even to have skill in using various teaching methods. The teacher must also understand some truths about how people learn and must know how to use these truths in planning and conducting classes. This chapter cannot replace a course in the psychology of education, but it will serve as a review of certain aspects of learning that undergird all teaching. Among the topics touched on here are generally accepted propositions about learning, types of learning, discovery learning, memory processes, and transfer of learning.

Propositions About Learning

Some propositions about learning are unique to a specific theory, such as conditioning theory, behaviorist theory, or Gestalt psychology, and do not receive widespread support from all learning theorists. Such propositions are of limited usefulness to the practicing teacher unless he or she subscribes to the particular theory. Other propositions are broad enough to be accepted by most learning theorists or psychologists and have been supported by sufficient research evidence to make them useful for all teachers, including nurse educators. Watson (1960) compiled a list of 50 learning propositions with which psychologists of any school would probably agree. Although his work was done a long time ago, the propositions still receive general acceptance by psychologists and educators today. Of the 50 propositions, those that apply to adult learners and are of importance to nurse educators are elaborated on in the following sections.

Reinforcement

1. "Behaviors which are rewarded (reinforced) are more likely to recur" (Watson, 1960; 254).

Positive feedback, or reward, is a powerful tool in the hands of a teacher. If a learner performs well in the clinical laboratory, and the teacher gives praise or a positive written evaluation, the learner's desirable behavior is more likely to be repeated than if the teacher had said or written nothing. In fact, absence of feedback is usually interpreted as negative feedback. If nothing is said about the clinical performance, the learner might well think that he or she did not do well that day.

Reward is just as important in the classroom as in the clinical laboratory. A student who raises an intelligent question in class and who is told that it is a good question, or is thanked for raising that issue, is more likely to ask questions in future classes. In grading papers, it is usually more valuable to write comments on the papers than to give only grades.

It is important to realize that what is rewarding for one learner may not be so for another. Student A may perceive a written comment on a paper as sufficient reward, Student B may require verbal praise as a reinforcer, and Student C may need no other reward than the satisfaction of a job well done. Although an instructor may not, in the course of a semester, learn exactly what kind of positive reinforcement each student needs, a general approach of positive verbal and written reward whenever possible and appropriate will serve to reinforce desirable behaviors for most students.

Immediate Feedback

2. "Reward (reinforcement), to be most effective in learning, must follow almost immediately after the desired behavior and be clearly connected with that behavior in the mind of the learner" (Watson, 1960; 254).

The student who gives a good answer to a question raised in the classroom should be given an immediate "Good" or "Right" rather than be told after class that it was a good answer. A learner in the clinical area should be given positive feedback at the time that something is done well; the instructor shouldn't wait until the end of the course to give the reward on the final evaluation.

The success of programmed instruction and computer-assisted

instruction can be attributed in part to the immediate feedback given to students. Immediate knowledge of success encourages the student to proceed and learn even more material.

Threats and Punishment

3.   "Threat and punishment have variable and uncertain effects upon learning; they may make the punished response more or less likely to recur; they may set up avoidance tendencies which prevent further learning" (Watson, 1960; 254).

Threats are frequently used in nursing education. Among the common ones are "If you don't turn in all three papers to me by Friday, you will fail the course" and "If you make one more mistake like that in the clinical area you will have to return to the college laboratory for more practice sessions." While these kinds of ultimatums are sometimes necessary to meet certain deadlines and constraints in a course, the effect on student learning is unpredictable. Instead of learning to hand papers in on time, for instance, the student may learn further avoidance techniques. The student who is punished by having to return to the college laboratory may or may not learn the skills presented there. If a student must return to the laboratory for remedial work, the instructor might try to present the situation as an opportunity to perfect skills in a less stressful environment, rather than as punishment or as banishment from the clinical area. Punishment may or may not eliminate unwanted behavior, but it does not help to move the student toward desirable behaviors—it takes reward to do that.

Threat and punishment are probably used more with beginning students than with RN learners, except in cases where a graduate has made many clinical errors. When this happens, the nurse must be made aware that his or her job is in jeopardy, but the emphasis should still be on the positive aspects of improvement of performance.

Practice

4.   "Sheer repetition without indications of improvement or any kind of reinforcement is a poor way to attempt to learn" (Watson, 1960; 254).

Every nursing instructor has had experience with learners who spend a great deal of time practicing skills in the college laboratory and yet still perform the skills incorrectly in the clinical area or on a skill test. That usually occurs because the learners have been practicing without reinforcement and develop poor habits, or at least fail to improve on each repetition. Thus, to be useful, practice must include feedback. This feedback can come through a laboratory instructor or a student aide in the lab or through use of audiovisual means such as videotaping with review. Practice without reinforcement also tends to be rather boring, and the nonmotivated student may simply stop practicing before the skill has truly been learned.

Stimulation

5. "Opportunity for fresh, novel, stimulating experience is a kind of reward which is quite effective in conditioning and learning" (Watson, 1960; 254).

Learning can be a reward in itself if the learning situation is interesting and novel. Too many laboratory and classroom experiences are boring and routine. Using a variety of teaching strategies such as role playing, brainstorming, and simulations can enliven the classroom and stimulate learning.

Motivation

6. "Learners progress in any area of learning only as far as they need to in order to achieve their purposes. Often they do only well enough to 'get by'; with increased motivation they improve" (Watson, 1960; 254).

We would all like to see nursing students achieve not just enough to "get by" but enough to excel and to have a positive effect on nursing care. Progression beyond the minimum may require added motivation and new goals.

Many students come into nursing with the goal of graduating so that they can support themselves by means of an interesting job. Some students express the desire for a field of work in which they can help people. Others are looking for the excitement of hospital life that they envision from having seen medical shows on television. Most of those in the first two groups probably work hard enough to graduate and achieve their goals. Those in the third group either quickly become disillusioned and leave the nursing program or develop a more realistic image of nursing and more realistic goals. In any case, even worthy goals are no guarantee that students will do any more than they absolutely have to in order to graduate. To work beyond this minimum effort, they must have some sort of motivation.

Some students have *intrinsic motivation* that helps them to excel. Intrinsic motives lie within the person and are the most effective type of motivation for significant learning and retention. Intrinsic motives include wanting to be the best at whatever job one undertakes and wanting to learn because learning brings its own satisfaction.

Teachers can also use *extrinsic motivation* to help students rise above mediocrity. Curiosity is a great motivator. The educator who can arouse students' curiosity in class or in the clinical laboratory and set them on the path to discovering the things they are curious about can help students want to do more than they absolutely have to do. Teachers can help students see the concrete rewards of providing quality nursing care: patients returned to a higher level of health than they would have achieved without help, patients who look to one as a caring and reliable professional, colleagues who value one's judgment and expertise, administrators that reward one with promotion.

Although educators would rather see students motivated intrinsically to do well, the fact is that most people need some extrinsic motivation, and as long as such motives are worthy, why not use them? Grades are undoubtedly extrinsic motivators. Fear of failure spurs students to study. However, frequent failure causes frustration and discouragement. A series of successes can be a powerful motivator to continue to do well, especially if there are occasional lapses; continuous success can sometimes interfere with motivation to learn if anxiety and fear of failure are forgotten (Bigge, 1971). Teachers can also use tests as extrinsic motivators for learning. For example, if an instructor wants students to learn application of principles and problem solving, her or his tests should be designed to test application and problem solving rather than memorization of facts; students will then be motivated to learn the material at the desired level.

Problem Solving

7. "Pupils 'think' when they encounter an obstacle, difficulty, puzzle or challenge in a course of action which interests them. The process of thinking involves designing and testing plausible solutions for the problem as understood by the thinker" (Watson, 1960; 255).

If nurses always dealt with routine patient situations and could apply proven nursing prescriptions to each situation, they would need to do little thinking or problem solving. But nursing is not that way. New, different, and puzzling problems frequently arise and require innovative solutions. Nursing students must be confronted with challenging assignments to enable them to learn to think as nurses.

When challenging classroom or clinical assignments are given, the teacher should guide the student when necessary but should not provide pat answers. Students need the practice of problem solving and must gain confidence in their ability to arrive at solutions. (Further information about problem solving is provided later in this chapter.)

Concepts

8. "The best way to help pupils form a general concept is to present the concept in numerous and varied specific situations, contrasting experiences with and without the desired concept, then to encourage precise formulations of the general idea and its application in situations different from those in which the concept was learned" (Watson, 1960; 255).

Nursing students are taught many concepts during their educational career. Take the concept of *priorities*. The best way to teach priorities might be to describe a patient care situation in which a staff nurse orders the priorities of care for the day. The instructor could describe the tasks and decisions that might face a head nurse and how he or she sets priorities in the work situation, describe an illness from a patient's perspective, and discuss how the patient might decide priority actions for getting well. The teacher could go on to contrast the care given by a nurse who successfully orders priorities with that of a nurse who does not, and then apply, or have the students apply, the concept of priorities to their own lives or to the work in the course.

Important concepts should not be left for students to haphazardly pick up as they go along. Concepts should be taught and taught well, so that students can use them as a sound base for further knowledge.

Frustration

2. "When children (or adults) experience too much frustration, their behavior ceases to be integrated, purposeful and rational. Blindly they act out their rage or discouragement or withdrawal.

The threshold of what is 'too much' varies; it is lowered by previous failures" (Watson, 1960; 255).

The student who is not doing well in a course may get caught up in a vicious cycle of frustration and failure. This scenario may develop in several ways. The student may blame the teacher and not take any responsibility for the failure. He or she may begin to feel worthless and defeated and withdraw from the course. Or the student may continue to try to succeed by using irrational methods such as staying up studying all night before an exam or frantically typing up all the class notes because he or she thinks that will help in learning the material.

I would like to be able to say that teachers never purposefully frustrate students, but I know that isn't the case. I have known nursing instructors who set out to cause a particular student to feel frustrated in class and the clinical laboratory so that the student, deemed unsuitable for nursing, will drop the course. There are more humane ways of steering students away from nursing than by causing them to become frustrated.

Students who are experiencing high levels of frustration need the teacher's help to reduce that frustration and prevent its ensuing irrational behavior. The teacher can help diagnose the student's problem, whether it is poor study habits, a weak theoretical background, insufficient time devoted to course work, or inability to cope with the level of work required. Whatever action is taken—remediation, schedule changes, or maybe even dropping the course—will help minimize frustration because student and teacher are working together to find the best solution to the problem.

Frustration may also be seen in new graduates who are experiencing reality shock. If not given support, they may lose self-confidence and quickly switch jobs. Professional guidance by staff development nurses can make all the difference in the outcome for these frustrated novices.

Peer Learning

10. "Pupils learn much from one another; those who have been together for years learn new material more easily from one of their own group than they do from strangers" (Watson, 1960; 256).

Students do learn from peers, and teachers should cultivate this source of education. Group projects, study groups, and demonstrations by students in the college laboratory are ways of taking advantage of learning from peers. Student tutors can also be used to help students in academic difficulty.

Techniques for Learning

11. "No school subjects are markedly superior to others for 'strengthening mental powers.' General improvement as a result of study of any subject depends on instruction designed to build up generalizations about principles, concept formation, and improvements of techniques of study, thinking, and communication" (Watson, 1960; 256).

Requiring students to take chemistry, microbiology, or calculus out of the belief that it will help them think more scientifically or will increase their memory abilities simply will not work. If science or math teachers spend time teaching students how to solve problems or analyze situations or how to apply learned principles in new situations, then "mental powers" may be strengthened. The same is true, however, for nursing courses. Although nursing content, like other course content, will not in itself improve mental skills, nursing professors may help students learn more effectively by helping them with study and memory techniques and with practice in problem solving and logical thinking.

Situational Learning

12. "What is learned is most likely to be available for use if it is learned in a situation much like that in which it is to be used and immediately preceding the time when it is needed. Learning in childhood, then forgetting, and then relearning when needed is not an efficient procedure" (Watson, 1960; 256).

Teaching material in the freshman year that will not be used until the senior year (or teaching class content in the first week of the semester that will not be used until the final week of clinical experience) is inefficient. Theory given in the classroom should be closely connected to clinical practice of that theory.

The proposition that students should learn subject matter in a situation much like that in which it will be used lends support to the teaching method of *simulation*. Written or laboratory simulations place the content in a clinical context that, although not as complex as the real world, helps learners see how the information they are learning affects a specific situation or is affected by the situation, and how the information actually fits into the real world setting. Learners are then more likely to recall and apply the content when practicing nursing.

Values and Attitudes

13. "Children (and adults even more) tend to select groups, reading matter, TV shows, and other influences which agree with their own opinions; they break off contact with contradictory views. Children remember new information which confirms their previous attitudes better than they remember new information which runs counter to their previous attitudes" (Watson, 1960; 256).

While nursing instructors usually have a general goal of socializing students into nursing and helping them form attitudes and values in keeping with the ethical and moral standards of the profession, they must remember that students enter the nursing program with values and attitudes that may contradict those of the faculty. The students may not be deeply affected by views that do not fit with their own unless instructors find means of modifying the original views held by the students. For example, some students may enter the program with little interest in or concern for the needs of the elderly patient. Lecture material about the needs and problems of the elderly may have little effect on the student unless he or she can first be brought to feel a certain empathy for the elderly and interest in them as a group. This doesn't mean that all students have to love geriatric nursing, but they should at least gain an appreciation of the special needs of that group.

Changing attitudes is not an easy task, but it is possible to do so with techniques such as providing students with positive clinical experiences with the elderly, using role playing and simulations in class, or assigning groups of students to work together on interesting assignments to uncover the problems or interests of the elderly and to suggest how nurses can improve the situation. The following chapters will provide some insight into teaching strategies that are helpful in changing attitudes.

Application of these thirteen generally accepted propositions of learning can help the teacher to be more effective in achieving the goals of instruction. They can also aid the educator in understanding why certain students act the way they do and why certain teaching strategies work in a particular situation while other strategies do not. For further explanation of the principles of learning, consult a text on educational psychology.

Types of Learning

Gagné, in a classic 1970 work titled *Conditions of Learning*, delineated eight types of learning. I will quickly describe all eight types and then will focus in more depth on the most complex type, problem solving.

Signal Learning

The first learning type is *signal learning*, or the conditioned response. On this simplest level of learning, the person develops a general diffuse reaction to a stimulus. For example, a nursing student may feel fear every time the term *skill test* is mentioned because he or she has felt fear whenever taking an actual skill test. Because of the association, just the words *skill test* are enough to evoke fear—they have become the signal that elicits the response.

Stimulus-Response Learning

Stimulus-response learning involves developing a voluntary response to a specific stimulus or combination of stimuli. An example of stimulus-response learning is the student nurse learning to monitor an intravenous infusion. Initially the instructor may tell the learner, "If you see that an intravenous infusion is not dripping, first open the clamp farther." This action may be demonstrated and reinforced in the clinical area. Eventually the learner responds automatically to an intravenous line that is not running by opening the clamp before doing anything else. This behavior can also occur at a higher conscious level of learning, but the simple, almost automatic muscular reaction of reaching out and opening the clamp can be a simple stimulus-response sequence.

Chaining

Chaining is the acquisition of a series of related conditioned responses or stimulus-response connections. After learning to open the clamp farther if an intravenous line is not dripping, the student nurse is taught that if opening the clamp is not successful, checking the line for a return blood flow is in order. This second step becomes another automatic response in a chain of responses.

Verbal Association

Verbal association is really a type of chaining and is easily recognizable in the process of learning medical terminology. A student already knows that the word *thermal* refers to temperature. The instructor introduces the word *hyperthermia* and its definition. The student recognizes that the syllable *therm* connects the two words and thus finds it easier to learn the new term because of a previous association.

Discrimination Learning

A great deal can be learned through forming large numbers of stimulus-response or verbal chains. However, the more new chains that are learned, the easier it is to forget previous chains. To learn and retain large numbers of chains, the person has to be able to discriminate among them. This process is called *discrimination learning*. For example, a student tries to learn a long list of drugs and their actions. Halfway down the list, the learning of new chains interferes with the memory for old ones. If the student can find a means of discriminating between the drugs, maybe finding something unique or noteworthy about each, retention will be increased.

Concept Learning

Concept learning is learning how to classify stimuli into groups represented by a common concept. Students enter college with a great deal of experience with concept learning. They have learned concepts ranging from *up* and *down* and *right* and *left* to *justice* and *democracy*. But they learn still newer concepts in the nursing curriculum. They learn a concept such as *asepsis,* first hearing what the word means, then having it pointed out to them in a variety of situations ranging from handwashing to sterile technique in the operating room. It may take a long time, but they will learn to identify the concept of asepsis in new situations and will be able to put the concept into use.

Rule Learning

A rule can be considered a chain of concepts or a relationship between concepts. A nursing student learns that to prevent a decubitus ulcer the patient must be turned, or if there is an open wound, sterile technique must be used. It is possible that a student may learn these statements simply as verbal chains and not understand or be able to apply the concepts. This happens, for example, when students memorize their notes for an exam but do not understand their application. True rule learning involves knowing each concept and being able to put relationships between concepts into use.

Problem Solving

Problem solving is the eighth and highest level of learning. To solve problems, the learner must have a clear idea of the problem or of the goal being sought and must be able to recall previously learned rules that relate to the situation. The next step is a thinking process in which the learner combines the recalled rules to form a new, higher-order rule that is then available for use in similar situations in the future. Therefore, a problem, once solved, theoretically will never be a problem again. The person will have only to recall the solution upon encountering that problem or a similar one.

Another way of viewing problem solving is as a process of formulating and testing hypotheses. The student, confronted with the problem, begins to formulate hypotheses, a process analogous to combining recalled rules to form a higher-order rule. Tentative solutions are mentally or actually planned and tested to see if they work, then modified as necessary (Houston, 1981).

An example of how nursing students use problem solving in the process of learning might be helpful at this point. Suppose a learner is planning care for a patient who has been stabilized after a myocardial infarction but is still on strict bedrest. As the instructor, you ask the learner how he or she is going to prevent muscle weakness in this patient yet also prevent strain on the heart. The problem has now been identified. The learner will recall rules that relate to exercise, muscle tone, and strength and will remember that passive isotonic exercise puts the least demands on the circulatory system, making it relatively safe for the stabilized myocardial infarction patient to maintain some muscle strength. The learner will then test the solution in actual practice. He or she has now learned a solution to this exact problem and related problems and will probably be able to recall the solution in future situations. If the learner had simply been told the solution, problem solving learning would not have taken place; the learner might not have truly understood the concepts involved and might not retain the information.

Bigge differentiates between "understanding-level" teaching and "memory-level" teaching. He states that "if understanding-level teaching is successful, students will know, in addition to the facts, the principles by which the facts are related; memory-level teaching tends to ignore principles, or at best handles them on such a superficial level that they have little meaning" (1971; 311). If students are to understand and retain information and have insight into problems, most of their nursing education should be at the rule-learning, problem-solving, and understanding levels.

You, as the teacher, play an important role in problem-solving learning. First, you can help the student to define the problem and the goal. You may simply state the problem or help the student put it into words by verbal coaching. You should be fairly certain at this point that the student has already learned the concepts and rules that will be needed to solve the problem. In the second step, you help the student recall the necessary rules by means of questions, suggestions, or demonstration. Students are learning a large number of rules and concepts in a short period of time and probably need help to select the rules that may apply to the problem situation.

Returning to the problem of the cardiac patient on strict bedrest, let me illustrate how the teacher could help the learner through the problem-solving process, allowing the learner to reach the solution:

Teacher: What is Mr. Davis's activity order?

Learner: He's on strict bedrest, but he can bathe and feed himself.

Teacher: Why is he on strict bedrest?

Learner: Because the doctor ordered it.

Teacher: I meant, why did the physician write that order?

Learner: I guess so that Mr. Davis's heart can rest.

Teacher: Good. There shouldn't be any strain on his heart muscle. But while his myocardium is resting, what is happening to the rest of the muscles in his body?

Learner: They're resting too—getting weak.

Teacher: Yes. Is there anything we can do to prevent the skeletal muscles from getting any weaker, yet not put strain on his heart muscle?

Learner: Maybe he could do isometric exercise—that doesn't cause much movement.

Teacher: It doesn't cause much movement, because the muscle fibers don't shorten, but it does cause other physiologic effects.

Learner: I remember now. Isometric exercise raises blood pressure.

Teacher: Right. It not only raises the blood pressure, it also increases cardiac output.

Learner: Well, we can't do that. (Pause) Could he do range of motion exercise?

Teacher: What kind of exercise is range of motion—what classification?

Learner: It's isotonic exercise. The muscles move and the fibers shorten.

Teacher: Yes, they move, but they actually require less oxygen than isometric exercise.

Learner: I guess Mr. Davis could do active range of motion of his arms because he is allowed to wash and feed himself. What about his legs?

Teacher: You can check with the physician about the extent of leg exercise Mr. Davis should start with.

In this example, the teacher led the learner through the problem-solving process, aiding in the recall of principles and rules, helping the student to think clearly and to arrive at a goal. Students who can recall principles and rules independently do not need this much guidance from the instructor in arriving at a solution.

Individual differences among students affect their ability to learn through problem solving (Gagné, 1970). A student who has learned a large repertoire of rules is more likely to have access to some rules that will apply to the situation at hand. But students also vary in their ability to recall those rules. Gagné also notes differences in *concept distinctiveness* among students; that is, some students are more able to select useful and relevant concepts that will help to define and solve the problem. Students may also differ in their ability to combine rules into hypotheses and to apply specific solutions to a general class of problems. These intellectual and creativity factors account for why some students do so well at problem-solving learning while others find it a struggle.

Discovery Learning

Educators and psychologists believe that problem-solving learning is closely allied to *guided discovery learning*, in which students are assisted in the process of discovering concepts, rules, and solutions, without information just being handed to them by the teacher.

Jerome Bruner, the outstanding leader in discovery learning, states that it includes "all forms of obtaining knowledge for oneself by the use of one's own mind" (1961; 124). This is a broad definition that includes two aspects of discovery learning, guided and unguided.

Unguided, or autonomous, discovery is the method of allowing students to pursue their own discoveries without assistance or direction from the teacher. This practice is rarely condoned by educators and is not considered appropriate in most classrooms. It is acceptable only if the purpose of the exercise is to teach students how to discover rather than to teach students prescribed subject material (Richards, 1973).

Guided discovery, on the other hand, is advocated by educators because it can be used to achieve many educational objectives. The guidance can consist of open-ended questions, hints, or directed questions. The direction (not answers) can be given by the teacher, by textbooks, or by programmed materials. Guidance reduces wasted time and increases the speed of learning (Entwistle, 1981).

Discovery learning may be accomplished through inductive or deductive methods. In *inductive* discovery, the teacher presents students with examples and data that they can analyze and manipulate in order to infer the general concept or principle. In *deductive* discovery, the teacher supplies students with concepts of some type and asks them to figure out dependent propositions. Of the two methods, the inductive approach is more widely used. In either case, the role of the teacher is to guide students into the correct line of questioning to make sure that their sequence of thinking is correct and that their conclusions are correct or compatible with known evidence.

Perhaps at this point it would be helpful to give some examples of situations in which the discovery method is used with children.

To teach the spelling rule "*i* before *e* except after *c*," most teachers would didactically tell students the rule. To teach this situation through discovery, the teacher would supply students with many words containing *ie* or *ei* and let them work with the words until they discover the rule (Chambers, 1971). In science, a student might be given the task of discovering the types of levers and how they function. The teacher would provide the equipment and allow the student to manipulate and experiment with the levers. Through careful questioning by the teacher, the student could come to actually see the meaning and use of levers and be able to reproduce this information at a later time (Mosston, 1972).

Benefits of Discovery Learning

The discovery method has certain advantages and disadvantages. Proponents believe that the greatest value of this method is that it promotes the habits of inquiry, autonomous thinking, and problem solving. (Discovery can be considered a broader topic than problem solving but is closely allied with it.) If we teach students how to inquire and when to inquire, we are providing them with an extremely useful and necessary skill. We cannot teach students everything we think they need to know by means of exposition and then expect them to know how to go beyond this and discover things for themselves. Students must be taught how to learn; if we want to produce independent thinkers, we must teach and foster independent thinking in the classroom and the laboratory.

A second advantage of discovery learning is that it increases student motivation and interest. A study done by Tamir and Goldminz (1974) supports the hypothesis that intrinsic motivation is a benefit of discovery learning. Students in the study felt that being confronted with a problem created a motivation to solve the problem; it became a personal challenge. Discovery learning arouses a student's curiosity, and curiosity is a great motivator.

Increased retention of learned material is a third advantage of discovery. Many studies have indicated that information learned through discovery is retained over a longer period of time than that learned didactically (Weisner, 1971). This effect is attributed to the fact that students are active participants in the learning process and invest part of themselves in the discovery. This benefit is supported by Tamir and Goldminz's (1974) finding that graduate students had a clear and detailed memory of subjects learned by discovery even as far back as elementary school.

A fourth benefit of discovery learning is *transfer of learning*, or application of current learning to future situations. (This concept is discussed in greater detail later in this chapter.) Studies done over the last 20 years suggest that discovery learning is more effective than traditional learning with regard to transfer of learning. By its very nature, discovery learning teaches for transfer. Students are taught to find relationships between data and situations, and they are given practice in applying already learned solutions to new and similar problems, all of which provides practice in transfer. Having basic nursing students and RN students discover concepts and generalizations that could be transferred to various clinical situations is an invaluable strategy.

Even those educators and psychologists who praise the discovery method admit that it has some decided disadvantages and drawbacks. From a practical and economic point of view, discovery learning is time consuming and expensive. It definitely takes longer for a student to discover something than for the teacher to give the answer. The investment is a sound one, however, if students can learn how to inquire and how to learn. In the clinical laboratory, discovery learning is appropriate and no more expensive than other approaches because the instructor is already working with a small group of students in an experiential setting.

Application to Nursing Education

Relatively little information about discovery learning has appeared in the nursing literature. Harms and McDonald (1966) described the inquiry method of teaching (discovery) as it was used in one baccalaureate program. The goal of their program was to help students develop skill in decision making and problem solving. They presented students with a problem and some facts and encouraged them to generate new ideas and solutions. This method was used during formal classes, in seminars, and in clinical settings.

In 1968 deTornyay studied the effectiveness of the discovery method in teaching student nurses to draw conclusions and generalizations about the concept of homeostasis. She found no significant difference in problem-solving skills between those taught by discovery and those taught by other means; both groups did equally well.

Bailey, McDonald, and Claus (1970) explored the effectiveness of the experimental curriculum at the University of California, San

Francisco, School of Nursing. This curriculum was developed to educate students to solve problems creatively, discovering solutions to problems rather than being told what solutions usually work. The researchers concluded that the curriculum was successful. The experimental group tested higher than the control group in verbal creativity, which the authors considered to be a factor necessary to creative nursing care.

The review of the nursing literature is not impressive; there is not much evidence, especially recent evidence, of the use or testing of discovery learning. The existing articles nevertheless show a concern for teaching nursing students independent, creative, problem-solving behavior.

Discovery learning could be incorporated into nursing education in a number of ways. The study of pathophysiology lends itself to this strategy. For example, students could be led to discover how ischemia occurs and how it manifests itself. They could investigate how vital signs are related to each other and why a change in one measurement accompanies changes in the other measurements.

Beginning students could be guided into discoveries about basic nursing care. Based on their science background, students could inquire into how decubitus ulcers develop and how they are cared for and treated. They should be able to discover what kind of nursing care should be given to an individual with dyspnea. At a higher level, graduate nurses could devise their own assessment scales and decide what they need to know to judge a client as being healthy. They could be encouraged to carry out nursing skills in new ways while still following the principles.

Whatever the subject matter, you as the teacher must foster divergent and creative thinking. You must be careful not to give too many answers when the student is expected to inquire on his or her own and not to give pat solutions and examples that will stifle the student's thinking. The discovery approach lends itself to seminar and small-group settings; it can be used naturally and productively in the clinical laboratory and in preconferences and postconferences.

Remembering and Forgetting

Studies have indicated that greater amounts of retention, and therefore less forgetting, can be expected when problem solving and discovery learning are used. The reasons behind these findings are of great interest and importance.

Take a look at Figure 2-1, a graph of a typical pattern of retention and forgetting. Lest you become too despondent after realizing the implications of this curve, let me point out that this type of curve usually refers to the learning of nonsense syllables or isolated facts. Little if any of this type of learning will be retained after a long interval. The learning of meaningful material presents another picture. Information that is meaningful and that is seriously studied may be retained very well (Gibson, 1980). Meaningful material consists of principles, rules, and generalizations that are applied in situations the student will encounter. It should be clear, then, why information learned through problem solving and discovery is retained much longer than isolated facts simply handed to the student.

Other factors that affect remembering and forgetting are the attitudes of the student toward the material, the amount of interference from other activities, and the degree to which the material has been learned (Gibson, 1980). As mentioned earlier in this chapter, students tend to remember information with which they agree and forget that with which they disagree. A study that supports this proposition was reported by Bigge (1971). In this research, students were divided into two groups, those with pro-communist attitudes and those with anti-communist attitudes. Both groups were given

Figure 2-1   **Typical Retention/Forgetting Curve**

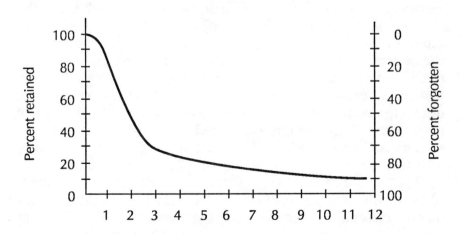

reading material that included pro- and anti-communist arguments. On a later memory test, the students with pro-communist sentiments remembered the pro-communist arguments best, while those with anti-communist opinions recalled the anti-communist arguments best.

Interference effects must also be considered. Previously learned items can interfere with present learning, and newly learned items can interfere with recall of past learning. For example, a student may have previously learned many medical terms and their definitions, but when he or she attempts to learn more terms within a short time, it seems as if the brain's memory banks are already full and will not accept any more terms. Or, the student may learn a host of new terms only to realize with dismay that he or she has forgotten the old terms.

A third factor that affects retention and forgetting is the degree to which the material is originally learned. Even information that is not essentially meaningful will be retained if it is studied in all seriousness and practiced and recalled periodically. Research has indicated that information is remembered for longer periods if it is studied and reviewed periodically rather than crammed into one session (Bigge, 1971; Garrison & Magoon, 1972). *Overlearning* also helps a person retain information. Overlearning is continued practice beyond the point of mastery. If a person learns how to perform a skill to the point of carrying it out correctly and smoothly but then continues to practice it until boredom sets in, the skill will be very resistant to extinction.

All these factors have obvious implications for developing effective study habits. Most experienced nursing educators can tell stories of students who were surprised at failing a test because they "studied so hard for it." Examining such students' study habits often reveals that they simply read and reread the class notes and the textbook or practiced a skill only once or twice because it seemed so easy and they had gotten it right the first time. Teachers have a responsibility to help students develop better study habits or to refer them to other professionals who can help them. Students need to learn the importance of spaced review versus cramming for an exam, of understanding notes and applying them versus simply reading them, and of overlearning through repeated practice.

The teacher can also assist students in retention of learning by planning for certain conditions. First, the teacher should make sure that the material to be covered is at the appropriate level. Then, the content should be presented in an organized manner, using a strategy that includes active participation of the student, if possible. If new learning is likely to interfere with already learned material, the teacher should spend extra time reinforcing both old and new concepts to help the student remember both. The instructor should not shy from using repetition to reinforce important material. It is helpful to summarize the content periodically, especially before beginning new content areas. When dealing with skill learning, the teacher should provide adequate time for student practice—supervised practice if possible. The teacher should also encourage overlearning of information and manual skills and the theoretical application of both to a variety of situations. Considering the tremendous amount of content that nursing students and RN learners are asked to learn, anything that teachers can do to enhance retention and prevent forgetting will be worthwhile.

Transfer of Learning

The goal of educators is not only to teach facts and information needed at the moment but also to develop capabilities and skills that will enable the learner to apply the learned information in future situations. Nurses must be able to apply classroom theory to an infinite variety of clinical situations. As noted earlier in this chapter, such carryover of information from the time and setting in which it was originally learned to new and different situations is called transfer of learning.

Types of Learning Transfer

We would like to think that all transfer of learning is positive—that is, that previously learned material augments learning or behavior in new circumstances. That is the case, for example, when a nursing student who has learned that the prefix *dys* means "difficult" or "painful" is later able to decipher the meaning of *dysuria* or *dyspnea* based on an understanding of the prefix. In *positive transfer*, learning is enhanced or accelerated by past learning. Unfortunately, transfer can also be negative. In *negative transfer*, past learning interferes with current learning. Negative transfer has occurred when a student who has learned that unconscious patients should be in a side-lying position with the bed flat to facilitate drainage of secretions places a head-injured unconsious patient in a side-lying, flat position, not considering the danger of increased intracranial pressure. In such a case, previously learned information has interfered with appropriate behavior in the new situation. Most of the time, with proper planning and the use of selected teaching methods, teachers can maximize positive transfer and prevent negative transfer.

According to Gagné (1970), transfer can also be classified as either lateral or vertical. *Lateral transfer* is generalizing the learned material to other situations of about the same level of complexity. For example, if a nursing student learns how to use the nursing process to develop a nursing care plan for a hypothetical patient described in class and then successfully writes a nursing care plan for a patient in the hospital who has different problems, lateral transfer has taken place. *Vertical transfer* occurs when capabilities learned at one level enhance learning of new, higher-level capabilities. A student who has taken physics and learned the material well may absorb information about orthopedic traction faster than a student who has not had the physics background. Both types of transfer can be facilitated by the teacher.

Maximizing Transfer

Three basic principles should be kept in mind regarding transfer of learning. First, transfer is most likely to take place when there are "identical elements" between the training and the transfer situations (Humphreys, 1974; 276). Thus, if you want students to solve problems in clinical situations, it would be best to teach them the process of problem solving in simulated clinical situations. Second, information taught in a meaningful way transfers more readily than information taught in a rote fashion (Humphreys, 1974). As already indicated, discovery learning transfers well because it is meaningful learning. Learned material that consists of principles, rationales, and generalizations is more likely to be transferred than relatively meaningless facts. Third, transfer does not take place unless the initial learning is sound. A learner who does not remember or who does not understand a body of knowledge obviously cannot transfer it. In general, the more a person knows about a given area, the more transfer that can take place (Houston, 1981).

To maximize transfer of learning, a teacher must plan for it, just as he or she plans to meet other course objectives. Here are some hints for doing such planning:

1. Analyze and formulate your objectives, and clarify which aspects of the course are necessary and desirable for transfer.

2. Select content that is most likely to be applicable in the student's future and plan teaching methods that will facilitate transfer (such as discussion, role playing, and problem solving in simulated situations).

3. Discuss with students the necessity for transfer and how to prepare for it.

4. Provide practice in transfer through simulations, projects, questions, and laboratory experience.

5. Perhaps most important, teach content in a meaningful way so that students can understand, manipulate, and apply the information.

Much of what is taught in nursing is transferable, and teachers can make more efficient use of teaching time if they emphasize transfer. A classic example of transferable content in nursing is the concept of asepsis. Instead of teaching particular aseptic practices involved in gloving, and later in changing a dressing, and later still in catheterization, why not first teach principles of asepsis, emphasizing full understanding of these principles, and immediately demonstrate use of these principles in a variety of situations, from gloving to wound irrigations, in each case pointing out the application of the principle? The students might not be required to remember all the steps of each procedure at the time but would see the applicability of the principles and would learn the possibilities of transfer. Future learning of aseptic procedures would be easier, and the students would have a good grasp of the concept of asepsis.

Inservice educators who are teaching a new skill, such as the use of a new infusion pump, should encourage transfer of knowledge. They can do so by referring to the basic principles of volume control and rate control that were learned previously and then pointing out how these same principles underlie the use of the new equipment.

All course planning must be done with transfer in mind if learners are to safely implement the theory with which they have been provided.

References

Baily JT, McDonald FJ, Claus KE: Evaluation of the development of creative behavior in an experimental nursing program. *Nurs Res* 1970; 19:100–107.

Bigge ML: *Learning Theories for Teachers*. Harper & Row, 1971.

Bruner JS: The act of discovery. *Harvard Educ Rev* 1961; 31:124–135.

Chambers DW: Putting down the discovery learning hypothesis. *Educ Tech* (Mar) 1971; 11:54–58.

deTornyay R: The effect of an experimental teaching strategy on problem solving abilities of sophomore nursing students. *Nurs Res* 1968; 17:108–113.

Entwistle NJ: *Styles of Learning and Teaching*. Wiley, 1981.

Gagné RM: *Conditions of Learning*. Holt, Rinehart and Winston, 1970.

Garrison KC, Magoon RA: *Educational Psychology*. Charles E Merrill, 1972.

Gibson JT: *Psychology for the Classroom* 2d ed. Prentice-Hall, 1980.

Harms M, McDonald F: The teaching-learning process. *Nurs Outlook*, 1966; 14:54–57.

Houston JP: *Fundamentals of Learning and Memory* 2d ed. Academic Press, 1981.

Humphreys LG: Transfer of training in general education. Pages 274–280 in: *Psychological Foundations of Education: Readings*. Goldberg ML, Werle M (editors). MSS Information Corporation, 1974.

Mosston M: *Teaching: From Command to Discovery*. Wadsworth, 1972.

Richards C: Third thoughts on discovery. *Educ Rev* 1973; 25:143–150.

Tamir P, Goldminz E: Discovery learning as viewed in retrospect by learners. *J College Science Teaching* 1974; 4:23–26.

Watson G: What psychology can we feel sure about? *Teachers College Record*, 1960; 61: 253–257.

Weisner C: Comparison of the effectiveness of discovery vs. didactic methods and teacher-guided vs. independent procedures in principle learning. *J Educ Res* 1971; 64; 217–219.

Chapter 3

Planning and Conducting Classes

The most formidable task a new teacher may face is the actual planning of classes. Even with a well-developed curriculum in place, the novice instructor has to decide:

What should I include in each class and what should I leave out?

What methods should I use in the classroom?

How do I know how long it will take to teach this amount of material?

How can I keep students interested and make sure that they learn?

It is not only new teachers who face such questions; we all have to deal with everyday planning of classes in such a way that they help meet curricular objectives, and individual student learning needs, while keeping ourselves stimulated even if we have taught the same information many times over. In this chapter I propose some helpful hints for both planning and conducting classes, based on research findings and on my own experience.

The Planning Sequence

Before you enter a classroom, you must do a tremendous amount of planning. You need to formulate objectives, select and organize content, choose teaching methods, and design assignments. You also have to decide how you are going to evaluate student learning. Ideally, you will complete all these steps before beginning to teach a course. In reality, when you are teaching for the first time, are teaching in a new institution, or are teaching a new course, time restraints may force you to continue with class preparation even after the course has begun. For your own sanity and for the sake of student learning, stay at least a few steps ahead of the students. However, even if your daily class preparation is ongoing, your planning of objectives, content, and evaluation methods should be completed before the course begins.

Formulating Objectives

You will need to formulate two levels of objectives: course objectives and objectives for each class. Some teachers also prefer to develop objectives for each unit within a course. All nurses today are familiar with objectives or goals in relation to patient care, and probably all have received reams of objectives written by professors in undergraduate and graduate courses. However, not all objectives are readable or useful. Some seem much too broad and some too specific. You should try to write objectives that have meaning not just for you but also for the students, who can use them to guide their studying.

The Value of Objectives   Why do you need objectives? First, you need them to guide your selection and handling of course materials. If your assignment is to teach a class on mental defense mechanisms, decide what you want the students to learn about such mechanisms before you outline your content. Once you have settled on your objectives, the content should flow naturally and easily from them.

Second, you need objectives to help you determine whether students have learned what you have tried to teach. You may have several vague ideas about what you would like students to know about defense mechanisms, but unless you have specific objectives, your evaluation of their learning may miss the mark. Your objectives should be specific enough that they enable you to know what the student will do, say, or think if he or she has learned this material.

Third, objectives are essential from the students' perspective. They need to know more about a course than they can get from a course description or a list of course content. They must be given objectives that communicate clearly what they will be expected to know and do with the course material. If tests are given in a course, the objectives should guide the students in their studying. For example, in a course (or unit) on psychological reactions to stress and illness, a session might be devoted to defense mechanisms. If the students have only a list of class topics, they will be unprepared for studying these mental mechanisms and will not know what material they will be held responsible for, unless the teacher spends a lot of time before each examination spelling out the plan of the test blueprint. Suppose, however, that students are provided with objectives such as these:

1. Explain the rationale for people's use of defense mechanisms.

2. Analyze in a given situation which defense mechanisms are being used by an individual.

In this case the students will know much more specifically what types of knowledge and skills are expected of them.

It is the teacher's responsibility to follow through and require students to demonstrate abilities that have been delineated in the objectives. Instructors who ignore their own course or class objectives when it comes time to evaluate students are generally regarded as unfair or as guilty of writing "tricky" exams or grading papers arbitrarily.

Types of Course Objectives   Objectives for an entire course are naturally much broader than class objectives. The number of course objectives usually varies from 5 to 15. The objectives are included in the course syllabus, along with the course description, course requirements, and reading list. They should also be discussed in the first class session so that students are immediately clear about what they will be expected to learn.

Course objectives are designed to be achievable by all students; they may be viewed as minimal competencies. It is the instructor's duty to plan learning experiences that will enable students to meet the objectives. If the objectives are unrealistic, either because the teacher's expectations are too high or because the needed learning experiences are inaccessible, they are worthless.

The types of learning encompassed in the course objectives may vary according to course content. Students may be expected to gain knowledge and comprehension, psychomotor skills, or new attitudes. One of the challenges of writing good course objectives is making them measurable. It is easy to measure knowledge and even comprehension, using various types of examinations or written or verbal assignments. Psychomotor skill objectives are probably the easiest to measure because students can be required to demonstrate their learning in some physical way. The difficulty comes with measuring affective objectives. You may want the student to gain an appreciation for the subject, to develop positive attitudes toward certain issues or groups, or to develop a greater understanding of an ethical issue. How can you measure this kind of learning—or can you even be assured that you can teach these types of learning?

Because it is difficult to measure affective objectives, many teachers avoid writing them. But without such objectives, the danger is that instructors will not try to teach affective issues. If they don't plan on teaching the ethical, attitudinal, and valuing aspects of a subject, these issues may simply get lost or will be learned haphazardly at best.

One key to writing affective objectives is to try to determine what measurable behaviors would indicate that a student has desirable attitudes or ethical standards. For example, you may want to instill the ethical imperative of confidentiality of communications between nurse and patient. Rather than writing an objective such as "Recognizes the importance of confidentiality in nurse-patient communication," which would be difficult to measure, you might substitute "Defends, in writing, the refusal of a nurse to divulge confidential information given by a patient" or "In a clinical situation does not discuss patient confidences with other patients, students, or staff." Although it is difficult to get the full flavor of the affective domain in a behavioral objective, it is better to try than to abandon the effort.

Writing such specific objectives as these last examples could lead to too long a list of course objectives. For that reason, some educators favor broad course objectives such as "Recognizes the importance of confidentiality in nurse-patient communication." Even though they are not concretely measurable, the implication is that they could be measured. The specific behavioral component of the objective can be left to class or unit objectives.

It is important to have objectives for each class session in which you meet with students. These objectives should have a narrow focus and behavioral format. The student's attention should, at the beginning of class, or at least the beginning of a unit of content, be drawn to what he or she is expected to learn by the end of the class or unit. Class objectives are usually few—only three to five per class session. They are invaluable in helping you prepare your content and select teaching methods and evaluation methods for the session. Class objectives may be written and handed out to students on a weekly basis or for units of content, or they may be presented verbally or on an overhead transparency at the beginning of a session.

Wording of Objectives   The actual wording of a behavioral objective is not crucial as long as it clearly and realistically describes the behavior to be learned. Some educators believe that an objective is incomplete unless it contains the behavior to be performed, the product of the performance that will be evaluated, and the conditions under which the performance will take place. By these standards, an objective might be written as "The student will explain the rationale for use of mental defense mechanisms by means of an in-class essay." Such detail is not always necessary and is possibly detrimental to student learning, because students might prepare specifically for this essay and neglect to read or study further information about the subject. Instead, the objective may be written in this way "The student will explain the rationale for use of mental defense mechanisms." It is then left to the teacher's discretion whether to evaluate learning with an essay that explains the general purpose of defense mechanisms or with a few multiple-choice questions that can elicit the student's knowledge of why certain mechanisms are used. The teacher may even choose to show a video simulation of people using defense mechanisms and have students explain what is going on.

Selecting Content

The general outlines of course content are usually prescribed by the curriculum of the school of nursing or by a hospital staff development department. Sometimes the only direction a teacher is given is the course description, but more often someone's files contain previous course outlines or course objectives to guide the instructor in deciding what to teach. But it is still left to the teacher's discretion to determine exactly what to include on a particular topic and what can safely be skipped over.

Let's imagine that you are responsible for teaching a course in physical assessment. You are handed a course description and a list of course objectives indicating that the students will perform and write a nursing history and complete a physical assessment of each system of the body. You want to start developing objectives and an outline of content for your first week of class. The topic is going to be "Why Nurses Learn to Do Physical Assessment." After you jot down that heading, your pen may come to a stop. How much information should you include , and how much detail should you go into? Several factors can guide your decisions. The first consideration is how much time you can devote to the topic. The content you select will vary greatly if you have 30 minutes as opposed to 60 minutes. The second factor is the kind of background students have. If they have completed their anatomy and physiology courses and have had an introductory course in the scope of nursing, you will obviously want to take advantage of that knowledge. If the students have already taken a clinical nursing course or if you are teaching RN learners, your approach may again be somewhat different. Third, if a textbook has already been selected for the course, its depth of content can give you some hints as to what you need to include.

Cramming too much information into a class session is one of the pitfalls that some teachers, especially new ones, fall into. Give yourself time to discuss the meaningfulness of the subject and cover the important points without getting bogged down in a lot of details that students will never remember after the exam anyway. Some research evidence indicates that when class content is too detailed, students do not perform as well on tests as they do when content is less detailed (Ryan, 1968). Obviously, details are sometimes important, but details such as dates and places when nurses first began performing physical assessments are something students could probably well do without. It is better to spend your time discussing broad related issues and concepts pertaining to the topic than to give lists of facts and dates that few practicing nurses would remember or ever use.

Organizing Content

The way in which class content is organized can make all the difference between sessions that are enjoyable and smooth running and those in which students are irritated and grumbling and the professor is appalled to realize (or maybe is ignorant of the fact) that the students are not following what is being taught.

When preparing for a course, you should first pay attention to the sequencing of course content, ensuring that it follows some logical direction. Then, when plotting specific sessions, you should consider the college calendar. Try to avoid placing important or sensitive material that will take more than one class session on days that will be split by a long weekend or a vacation. It is also a good idea not to plan to teach any crucial material on the day before a vacation or on the last day of class before graduation. The best teacher in the world may not be able to rise above the restlessness that besets students around these times.

Allow for some flexibility in the class schedule. There is such a thing as being too rigid in adhering to a schedule. If you are working under the pressure of having to complete topic A on Monday so that you can start topic B on Wednesday, you may have to cut off valuable class discussion or ignore some profitable side issues raised by students. Although it is desirable to follow a planned schedule, especially if it is written and handed out to the students, some leeway must be allowed.

The organization of each class session is important to student learning and satisfaction. Lectures, especially, need to be organized. Sharing class objectives with the group sets the stage for an organized lecture. You can indicate, in the progress of your lecture, the headings and subheadings under which you are discussing the subject of the day. Nothing is more distressing than trying to take notes from a lecturer who skips all over a topic with no apparent rhyme or reason. I still retain a vivid memory of a professor who taught one of my research courses. In the space of a 2-hour class, this teacher would flit from random sampling to reliability and validity to correlation theory and back to sampling again, apparently unaware that the students were bewildered. We clung to the textbook as a lifeline for the whole course in order to keep our heads above water and make sense of the research process. If you are in any doubt about the organization of your lectures, you can have a colleague sit in on a class and critique that aspect of it, or you can tape the class and attempt to take notes on the lecture while playing it back. The results should be enlightening.

It is not only lectures that need to be organized. Discussions, role playing, and computer applications all need structure and organization if learning is to proceed smoothly. In a research course, I taught one class in which I used a computer program on statistics. The class began in the regular classroom, then moved to a nearby computer lab, and then returned to the original classroom. The moving alone necessitated planning and organization. The content also required strict organization lest the class disintegrate into a session of computer games. I began by giving the objectives for the day, then reviewed the particular statistical tests we were going to use on the computer program and handed out some raw data (in simulated situation form) that the students would run on the computer. When we went to the computer lab, the challenge was to achieve a balance between letting students work at their own pace (in small groups) and maintaining organization by helping each group run the program and the printout and understand what they were doing. On our return to the classroom, students had many questions. I attempted to organize my responses by fielding questions pertaining to one aspect of the process at a time. I finished with a summary of how to interpret the printouts. So you see, organization is important to any class session, regardless of methods used.

Selecting Methods

Deciding which teaching method to use, given the wide assortment available, is not easy. Which method is the best for teaching a certain body of information? Many factors should be considered.

Factors Affecting Choice of Method   First, the selection depends on the type of learning you are trying to achieve. If you want to present facts and rules, a lecture with handouts may be appropriate. If you want to mold attitudes, discussion or role playing may work the best. If your goal is to motivate students, gaming would be a good choice. If students need to learn a great deal of material in a short period of time, the best approach might be computer-assisted instruction or programmed learning. If you want to encourage creativity and problem-solving skills, your best approach would be discovery methods or individual projects. Different teaching strategies can yield different outcomes; you have to be clear about your goals for learning if you are to choose an appropriate method.

Course content also dictates methodology to some extent. A class on isolation technique may be effectively taught by demonstration, computer simulation, or hands-on practice but would be poorly taught by means of debate. The ethical aspects of euthanasia could be handled nicely in a seminar discussion or with a videotape and discussion but would not be taught as effectively by programmed instruction. Because nursing is a practice discipline, a lot of the learning should be active learning; that is, the student should be an active participant in the learning process. The teaching methods selected should therefore emphasize student activity:

discussion, debate, responses to case studies and simulations, role playing, computer use, and so on. Overdependence on lecture is indefensible in teaching material for a practice profession.

Choice of teaching method also depends on the abilities and interests of the teacher. From your experiences as a student you have probably developed some prejudices about teaching strategies. You may have hated audiotapes or debates as a student and will most likely not feel eager to use these methods when you teach. On the other hand, you may have learned a great deal from filmstrips and simulations and feel inclined to include them in your repertoire of methods. As you begin to use various methods, you will find that you feel comfortable using some and not others. Every teacher should capitalize on personal strengths and use those methods that are compatible with his or her personality and teaching style. At the same time, however, the teacher should keep an open mind about new methodologies and have the courage to try and persevere with new techniques.

Compatibility between teachers and teaching methods is important, but so is compatibility between students and teaching methods. You have to know the capabilities of your students. A class with many "weak" students requires different approaches than a class with mostly "superior" students. A weak group may need more structure and guidance than an intellectually strong group. For example, a class with a majority of students who are less intellectually gifted may need lectures and computer tutorials and audiovisual supplements. A superior class may learn better from Socratic questioning or from problem-solving simulations. Different classes also have different motivation levels, which may require changes in strategy. If all students have to meet the same objectives, you must be flexible about how you are going to help move them toward this goal. (Later in this chapter we will look further into individual learning styles.)

Another factor that influences the selection of teaching methods is the number of students in the class. Having 15 students versus 60 will obviously affect teaching strategies. Large groups lend themselves to lectures, movies, or possible case studies. With small groups, discussions, role playing, and videotapes can be more effective.

Finally, a teacher's instructional options are limited to the resources available in the institution. Classroom size, furniture, lighting, and especially availability of equipment such as projectors, screens, and computers all determine which strategies may be used.

Effectiveness of Various Methods   Research should shed some light on the superiority of some teaching methods over others, and in some respects it does. However, the findings depend greatly on the outcome criteria (dependent variables) used in the various studies. When the outcome is the acquisition of information, performance is about the same for all methods (Gage, 1976). But when the outcome being measured is problem solving ability, time saved in learning, or transfer of learning abilities, some methods prove to be better than others. (Research related to each teaching strategy will be covered in following chapters.) So, it would be inappropriate to claim that any one method is superior to another without asking, "Superior in which regard?"

Most methodology research has compared some "new" method against "traditional" methods. Comparing gaming to lectures would be a typical example. As McKeachie (1969) points out, the fact that a new or experimental method is being used lends excitement to the study, making it difficult to separate the effects of the emotional reaction from the actual learning effects of the new method. Whether on the part of the instructor or the students, the excitement about the method can affect the study.

Another extraneous variable that needs to be considered in evaluating the results of methodology comparison studies is that it may be the same teacher who uses both methods. That is, the same instructor may use gaming with the experimental group and lecture with the control group. The problem in this case is that the personality, style, and approach of the instructor can play a significant role in the success of a particular teaching method; some personality styles work well with some methods but not others. Therefore, as with any research, the results must be weighed carefully in light of the design and procedures. Full confidence should be placed only in results that have been replicated and confirmed.

Choosing a Textbook

For most nursing courses a textbook is a necessity, not an option. It would be difficult in a medical/surgical nursing course or parent/child nursing course to bypass a textbook and use just reading assignments from periodicals, because you would have to require so many readings as to be impractical. The amount of time and money that it would take for students to photocopy all of the required readings might be a real imposition, and copying articles yourself and distributing them to students violates copyright laws. There may be some courses, such as current issues, in which you might dispense with a textbook, but you should first make sure that there is no appropriate textbook on the market.

Many considerations should guide you when choosing a textbook. Talk to publishers' representatives or call publishers for review copies of likely texts so that you can examine them at some length in order to make the right decision. As Eble states, the most important consideration in choosing texts is "whether students are likely to read them, work with them, and learn from them" (1976; 86). Try to put yourself in the students' position and realistically decide from the outset whether they can and will use a particular book. If students see the text as superfluous and not central to the course, if they know they can get away without reading the text and still do fairly well in the course, or if they find the text too difficult or boring, they won't use it or learn from it. A lot depends not just on the appearance, writing style, or contents of the text but on the use the teacher makes of it, which I will discuss later.

The first step in examining a textbook is to read the preface. The preface is the author's description of what the book is all about, its general objectives, the types of students who can use it, and its intended use. This is all valuable information, and if a preface is done well, you can tell immediately whether the book's approach is appropriate to your needs (Parsons & O'Shea, 1986). Second, look at the table of contents to see how closely the content mirrors the content of your course. You may not always find an exact fit with your course, but you should be able to find at least one text that comes pretty close. You can supplement the text with some outside readings if you wish, and you can always leave out some of the text material.

By the time you have looked at the preface and table of contents, you should have a fairly good idea about whether the book is compatible with the philosophy and objectives of the school's curriculum and the objectives of your course. Further examination of chapter content will confirm your opinion. Look at a few of the chapters in depth. If you examine topics that you know a lot about, you can gauge the accuracy, currency, and depth of content. If all of the vital information is acceptable, read the chapter for clarity and style. Will the material be understandable to the novice, and will it hold his or her interest?

Next examine the book's appearance. Is the print easy to read and are the diagrams or charts easy to follow? Is the paper heavy enough that print does not show through the pages (Parsons & O'Shea, 1986)? Studies that have attempted to determine optimum print styles and sizes and line lengths have revealed a wide margin of acceptability and clarity. There is no one best type or size of print (Brown, Lewis & Harcleroad, 1969). However, if you find the print or line spacing unacceptable, many other readers will, too. Parsons and O'Shea state that "an attractive, easily understood, accurate textbook can be a servant in the finest sense" (1986; 344). The converse is also true, however. An unattractive, overly difficult, or inaccurate textbook serves little purpose except to forge negative attitudes in students and make teaching more difficult.

Another important factor to consider before selecting a textbook is the way in which the book will be used. Some instructors prefer a comprehensive, in-depth text from which they will choose topics for discussion or application. The student will not only use the text to prepare for class but will presumably save the book as a reference for the future. Other teachers prefer books that cover broad topics in less detail. Their class presentations are then built around adding depth and detail to those topics. The success of the chosen book and of the method used often depends on the abilities of the students, however. Less bright and less motivated students might do better with a more simplistic text that is further explicated in class.

The size of a book should also be a consideration. Many nursing texts today are so large and heavy that it would be ridiculous to expect students to carry them to class. If you plan to use a book in class, you should select a lighter volume. If the book is to be kept at home only for reading and study, size may not be a drawback.

The cost of textbooks is another practical issue. Instructors should be conservative with students' money and should find out the cost of the texts under consideration. If two books are nearly equal in all other respects, why not select the less expensive one? Cost should also be kept in mind when considering the value of supplementary books such as workbooks and study guides. Will they really be used? Keep in mind that students aren't usually buying books for only your course. They may be required to purchase books for four or five courses in one semester.

Just as important as the selection of a textbook is the way in which it will be used. Handing out a course syllabus that contains all of the reading assignments for the semester and then never referring to them again does not seem to be a justifiable procedure. Whether or not the instructor holds students responsible for the text material on examinations, he or she has not used the text in a meaningful way.

The teacher's goal should be to ensure that students indeed do the reading and understand the information they have read. Just testing the students on textbook material is not enough to meet that goal. The teacher also has to direct students in what to read for and should plan to use the information in some way. Instructors can take several approaches toward reading assignments. A common approach is to assign the pages for homework, assume the students have read the material and understand it, and carry on the next day's class as if the students have all this information mentally digested, catalogued, and stored for future use. Other instructors assume that few people have read or understood the assigned reading, so they rehash it all in class, which simply serves to reinforce the nonreading behavior. A third approach is to plan to use the information from assigned reading as a basis for classroom discussion. However, what often happens is that just a few of the students have read or understood the material, so they do all the discussing while the others vegetate or try to catch on. Finally, some instructors do the assigned reading themselves, make some notes about what to have the students focus on, and explain to students in advance how they should read the material and how it will be used in class. Gallo and Gallo (1974) refer to this last approach as *guided reading*.

Guided reading, Gallo and Gallo contend, will help keep students from underlining everything in the book, trying to memorize all the facts, or getting so bogged down in the overwhelming mass of information that they just give up and close the book. Students should read the assignment knowing what they should be focusing on, what they should get out of the assignment, and how the information will blend with class material. For example, an instructor may assign 15 pages of reading related to myocardial infarction. He or she tells the students to pay special attention to risk factors, because a preventive teaching plan will be formulated in class the next day, and to come prepared with any questions about the pathophysiologic process, which will be briefly outlined in class. This kind of direction will help many students learn from the reading assignment.

If a textbook closely parallels course content, the teacher can build on its foundation by discussing certain aspects of it in class and by using it as a basis for questioning, debate, role playing, and so on. By no means should the instructor merely repeat the text in a lecture. Lectures could be used to supplement a text that is not comprehensive or to provide differing viewpoints from the book. Creative use of a textbook is one of the challenges of teaching.

Planning Assignments

No less challenging is planning assignments other than textbook reading. Some courses may require only reading assignments; other courses have objectives that can be met only by other means.

One of the favorite teaching devices is the term paper, sometimes disguised as the topic paper, research paper, or position paper. Such papers are frequently assigned in introductory nursing courses, current issues courses, or professional theory courses. The standard term paper, usually 10–15 pages long, in which a student must research a topic and write it up in "scholarly form" with full documentation, is rarely appropriate or necessary. What does a teacher expect the student to learn from such an assignment—how to write a scholarly paper? how to organize one's thoughts? how to think analytically? how to find answers to questions and solutions to problems? Few of these goals are actually met by term-paper writing in a nursing course. What actually occurs is that the student learns a great deal about one topic (which may or may not have later usefulness), learns to get someone else to edit and type the paper, or may even learn how to buy a paper on the black market. There are better ways to meet the desired objectives.

If you want to see whether students can think analytically, assign a short essay in which they have to analyze a particular patient problem or an issue related to the course. This kind of assignment forces students to use their own analytical powers and not just rephrase someone else's ideas from the literature. If you want to test students' ability to use resources to answer specific questions, ask them the questions, let them investigate the answers, and have them write up the answers in a short paper. You might even ask students to write lists of pertinent questions that need answers.

There are other types of creative yet worthy assignments. Students could be asked to devise assessment forms or patient teaching materials. They could be asked to solve a problem in the real world of nursing and report on the solution. They could do personal interviews, formulate ideas for research, or keep logs and journals. Countless types of assignments are available that would help achieve course objectives and yet not involve a lot of busywork and repetition.

It is important to keep the students' workload in mind when designing assignments. Students may be carrying 15–18 credits. If for each 3-credit course they have to write a term paper plus keep up with readings and examinations, they probably live in stress and anxiety for the whole semester. Every teacher knows, but many forget, how long it takes to write a good 10- to 15-page paper. It's impossible for most students to produce more than one good paper per semester along with the rest of their workload. Even if you give short assignments, keep in mind how much time it will take the average student to complete them, and adjust the workload accordingly.

Some instructors see group projects as the solution to the workload problem. Group projects can provide useful learning experiences, but they are also time consuming and difficult to conduct. The group has to meet, often at inconvenient times, and group process does not always move smoothly. One group project per semester is probably enough for a student. Nursing faculty have no influence over what nonnursing faculty are assigning, but they can arrange within the nursing department to keep assignments equitable.

Nursing care plans are an indispensable part of the nursing instructor's assignments. Care plans need to be written for most clinical courses, but they are sometimes misused and abused. The objectives of preparing care plans should be clear in the instructor's mind. Will students be writing them as a means of learning the nursing process? planning care for an assigned patient? learning about typical nursing diagnoses and related nursing care? All three objectives can be met by writing care plans, but the types and size of the care plans may vary.

Beginning students who are learning the nursing process need to write simple, short care plans on simulated or real patient situations. They can learn the process without writing comprehensive, lengthy plans. If the student's goal is to write a plan of care for a particular patient, it will vary in length and comprehensiveness. For example, a "working" care plan that has to be devised every week in order to provide safe care should be as short as possible, maybe in Kardex form. Occasionally the teacher may be justified in asking students to enlarge these working care plans to include scientific rationale and documentation. When care plans become term-paper length, they are really case studies, and it's time for the teacher to look at his or her objectives to see whether the assignment is reasonable and necessary. It might be more appropriate for the student to write an in-depth assessment rather than a full care plan. Care plans written for the purpose of learning about typical nursing diagnoses and related nursing care are redundant in today's nursing world. There are published manuals of standard nursing care plans that can be incorporated in class content if desired.

Whatever the assignment for a course, it is the teacher's responsibility to read all student work carefully and soon after it has been handed in. Student papers should receive not only a grade but comments as well. If the teacher weighs his or her own workload when planning assignments, student work can be given due attention and returned promptly. Barring unforeseen eventualities, at the end of the course no teacher should have piles of papers still to be graded that have to be mailed to the students after the term is over. At that point feedback on assignments is no longer a learning experience.

Creating Examinations

Papers and similar assignments are not only learning experiences but also methods of evaluating learning. Examinations of one type or another are also important ways of assessing learning.

Good tests are devised after careful thought and planning, either before a course begins or at least well before examination time. They should test the achievement of course and class objectives logically and systematically. As we shall see shortly, good exam planning involves some type of test blueprint or table of specifications. A blueprint spells out the content (behaviors, objectives) and the level of knowledge to be tested.

It is helpful to use Bloom's (1984) taxonomy of educational objectives in testing levels of knowledge. Bloom identified three learning domains: cognitive, psychomotor, and affective. In the cognitive domain, he rated knowing on six levels, from *knowledge* (at the lowest level) to *comprehension, application, analysis, synthesis,* and finally *evaluation* (at the highest level). In any field of learning, but especially in a practice profession like nursing, test questions must be heavily weighted at the higher levels of knowing. It is not enough for a nursing student to be able to recall and understand facts (knowledge and comprehension levels); to be a problem-solving, analytically thinking professional, the individual must also be able to demonstrate abilities at the four highest levels of knowing.

Examination questions at the application level test the student's ability to use information learned in class in a new or concrete situation. At the analysis and synthesis levels, learners weigh the value or veracity of information, determine how much certain facts contribute to certain situations, and pull information together to arrive at a course of action or a conclusion. Evaluation questions require the student to judge whether certain data or courses of action are helpful, whether they solve the problem presented, and whether the given actions are appropriate.

Every test should be viewed as a sampling process. That is, out of the universe of facts, skills, and understandings that learners are supposed to gain in a course, an examination can test only a small portion. The teacher must decide how large the sample should be and what information deserves to be sampled. Performance on this sample of test items implies a similar grasp of the whole body of information taught. The problem, of course, is in selecting or creating a representative sample. A *test blueprint* aids in systematically planning the sample.

The blueprint or table of specifications can be highly specific or rather general, according to a teacher's preference. At the very least, it should contain the content or objectives to be measured, the levels of knowledge that will be tested, and the numbers of questions devoted to each area. It is also possible to include the types of questions that will be asked. Figure 3-1 is an example of a general test blueprint for a 50-question examination on oxygenation. The numbers of questions devoted to each box in the blueprint should depend on the time and emphasis given to that area of content in class or in reading assignments.

Deciding on the number of items to include on a test depends on such factors as amount of material taught, the type of test items used, and the amount of time available for testing. In general, the larger the sample, the more reliable the test. If you develop a blueprint and find that because of time constraints you can include only one or two items for each content area or objective, you may have to give more frequent tests (Gronlund, 1976).

The types of test questions that can be used are undoubtedly familiar to you. They include true/false questions, matching items, multiple-choice questions, short-answer questions, and essays. Examinations may consist of a single type of question or a combination of types, as long as the objectives are being measured at the desired levels of learning.

Developing good test questions is an art as well as a science and cannot be fully taught in a single chapter of a text such as this.

Figure 3-1   **Test Blueprint for Unit on Oxygenation**

CONTENT	LEVEL OF KNOWING				
	Knowledge/ Comprehension	Application	Analysis/ Synthesis	Evaluation	Total Items
Principles	2	2	2		6
Factors affecting	3	3	4		10
Pathophysiology	3	3	4		10
Assessment	1	3	4	2	10
Nursing measures		3	3	4	10
Evaluation of care		1	1	2	4
Total items	9	15	18	8	50

However, I will make some comments about the usefulness of each type of question and give some examples. Skill in writing test items can be developed in graduate courses or inservice courses in evaluation or by reading and applying information from test and measurement textbooks. However, keep in mind that it *is* a skill that needs to be learned and developed and will not magically appear overnight.

True/False Questions   True/false questions are designed to test a student's ability to identify the correctness of statements of fact or principle. True/false items are limited to testing the lowest levels of knowing, knowledge and comprehension, and tell the teacher only that the student knows that the statement is correct or incorrect but not whether he or she knows why it is correct or incorrect. There is also a 50/50 chance that the student has guessed the right answer. Teachers sometimes favor this type of question because it is relatively easy to write and to grade. Nursing exams, however, should contain few true/false questions.

When writing true/false items, make sure that you word the statement so that it is clearly true or false. For example:

> (T F) Diabetics who test their blood sugar four times a day
> have fewer complications than those who don't.

The answer to this question is "True" in many cases but "False" in others. Students would probably label this a tricky question. To make this question unequivocally "True," it should be worded

> (T F) Type I diabetics who test their blood sugar four
> times a day and take appropriate insulin have fewer com-
> plications than those who don't.

The rewording makes this item longer than desirable. If a true/false item gets too long, it might be better to use another type of question.

Avoid including terms like *always* or *never* in true/false questions. Test-wise people know that items with these qualifiers are likely to be false. Equally avoid qualifiers such as *sometimes* and *frequently* because they are open to interpretation by the reader.

Matching Questions   Matching questions test knowledge, the lowest level of knowing. They are useful in discovering the student's ability to recall the memorized relationship between two things, such as dates and events, structures and functions, medical symbols and their meaning, and terms and definitions. Again, because they are easy to construct and because they test a lot of information in a compact way, matching questions are popular among instructors, but this method should be used sparingly.

The two lists of items to be matched should be approximately the same length, with one or two extra options so that the learner cannot answer just by process of elimination. All items in the list should be homogeneous—all related to one topic or concept. Matching questions are usually set up in the following way:

> Match the abbreviation on the left to its meaning on
> the right. Place the appropriate letter in the space in front
> of the abbreviation.

_____ 1. a.c.   A. of each
_____ 2. c̄   B. without
_____ 3. gtt.   C. before meals
_____ 4. p.o.   D. drops
_____ 5. Q.h.   E. with
_____ 6. s̄   F. every hour
                 G. by mouth

The instructions can also indicate whether an option can be used more than once.

Double matching items can also be designed to increase the level of difficulty, as in the following (Carlson, 1985; 27):

> In the spaces on the left place the letters A, M, or H to identify the measurement system in which the abbreviation belongs. In the spaces on the right, place the letter of the accepted equivalent.

A = apothecaries'   a. 15 gr
M = metric   b. 1000 cc
H = household   c. 4 cc
                     d. 100 Gm
                     e. 30 cc
                     f. 15 cc
                     g. 2.2 lb
                     h. 4 dr

_____ 1. dr _____
_____ 2. oz _____
_____ 3. T   _____
_____ 4. Kg _____
_____ 5. L   _____
_____ 6. Gm _____

The level of difficulty can also be increased by lengthening the lists of items.

Multiple-Choice Questions   Nursing instructors rely heavily on multiple-choice questions for at least two reasons. First, the national licensing exams are written in this form, and teachers like to think that giving students lots of practice in answering multiple-choice questions will increase their chances of passing their state boards. Logically this seems to make sense, although I don't think it has been scientifically tested. Second, the multiple-choice format is flexible and can measure any level of learning (although as with any written test, it can measure only what a student knows, not what he or she would actually do in a nursing situation). It is easiest to write multiple-choice questions at the knowledge and comprehension levels, but it is possible, with practice, to write good questions at higher levels, such as application or evaluation. To demonstrate the differences, here are three questions, the first testing comprehension, the second application, and the third evaluation:

1. Which parameter is it most important for a nurse to report when implementing postural drainage?
   a. Frequency of oral hygiene.
   b. Number of times the patient coughed.
   c. Amount of sputum expectorated.
   d. Change in respiratory depth.

2. An immobilized alert patient is developing atelectasis. What should the nurse do first with this patient?
   a. Oral suctioning.
   b. Postural drainage.
   c. Pursed-lip breathing.
   d. Coughing and deep breathing.

3. An orthopneic patient is placed in high Fowler's position. What data would indicate the need to reassess the situation and maybe reposition the patient?
   a. Coughing and expectoration.
   b. Inability to rest.
   c. Decreased use of accessory muscles.
   d. Increased chest expansion.

Questions such as these test the intended level of knowing only if the exact information in the question has *not* already been taught in class. For example, if a teacher who taught that patients developing atelectasis should benefit from coughing and deep breathing but not from suctioning, postural drainage, or pursed-lip breathing were to use the second question on the exam, the item would be

testing recall of information—the knowledge level—not application. Because only the teacher knows what was taught and how it
was presented, it is only he or she who can determine for sure what
level of knowing the questions are really testing.

A multiple-choice question has two parts. The question itself is
called the *stem*. The possible answers or solutions that follow are
called the *options*. The correct option is termed the *answer* and the
incorrect options are called *distractors*. The stem can be worded as a
question or as an incomplete statement. Beginning item writers
may find it easier to write actual questions. In either case, the stem
should clearly state the problem and make sense in itself without
the reader having to look at the options to find out what is being
asked.

Here is an example of a correct stem worded as a question:

> Which phrase best defines atelectasis?
> a.   A collapse in a portion of a lung.
> b.   Fluid in the lung.
> c.   Fluid in the pleural space.
> d.   Outpouchings in the bronchial walls.

Here is a correct stem written as an incomplete statement:

> Atelectasis can best be defined as
> a.   a collapse in a portion of a lung.
> b.   fluid in the lung.
> c.   fluid in the pleural space.
> d.   outpouchings in the bronchial walls.

The stem should be clearly worded and not so long that the student
gets lost. The stem should include any words that might be redundant in the options. For example, if each option starts with "It
is a . . ." it would be better to put those words in the stem.

Negatively stated stems should be avoided unless they test
important points (Gronlund, 1976). Negative terms in the stem
tend to make questions more confusing. A question such as "Which
phrase does not define atelectasis?" would be poor because of the
focus on the negative. What would be the point of asking students
to focus on an incorrect definition? It would make sense, though, to
ask a negative question if it were important for a nurse *not* to do
something. For instance:

To prevent infection when inserting an intravenous catheter, a nurse should never . . .

Another way to handle negative questions is to write them in the "except" format, such as:

> All of these statements define atelectasis EXCEPT . . .

Although these kinds of questions are not recommended, it may be difficult to test some material without resorting to them at times. When they are used, the word *except* should be placed near the end of the stem and should be capitalized or underlined.

The number of options that follow the stem may vary. There is no magic in having four options, although that is the usual pattern. Three options are acceptable, as are five (Hills, 1981). The problem with four or five options is that it is difficult to formulate three or four plausible distractors. There should be only one right or best answer.

The distractors should be realistic. They are most attractive when they are based on common misconceptions that learners have about the topic. Nonsense distractors should never be used, and *all of the above* or *none of the above* should be used sparingly. *All of the above* may be used to increase the difficulty of the item. *None of the above* should be used only in cases similar to those calling for a negative stem, in which it is important for the student to know that avoiding certain practices or procedures is crucial (Gronlund, 1976).

A few more rules govern the writing of options. First, they should be grammatically consistent with the stem, both to use good style and to avoid giving unwanted clues. Too often inconsistency occurs only in the distractors, leaving the answer standing out as clearly right because it fits best grammatically (Gronlund, 1976).

Here is an example of a grammatically inconsistent item:

> The presence of "moderate" acetone in a patient's urine indicates that
>
> a.   fats are being burned for energy.
> b.   when blood sugar is very high.
> c.   ACTH levels are sometimes elevated.
> d.   it means protein is being metabolized.

Here is the same item made grammatically consistent:

The presence of "moderate" acetone in a patient's urine indicates that
a. fats are being burned for energy.
b. blood sugar is very high.
c. ACTH levels are elevated.
d. protein is being metabolized.

A second rule is that options should be fairly short and about the same length. It is easy to fall into the trap of making the correct answer longer than the distractors to include enough information to make sure that it is clearly true. If you have to write a longer answer, increase the length of the distractors as well. Options should also be placed in logical order if one exists, such as increasing or decreasing numbers or alphabetized terms.

Third, avoid the use of qualifying words, sometimes called *specific determiners*, that give clues to the reader (Hills, 1981). People who become test wise know that words like *all*, *always*, and *never* in the options probably indicate false statements, whereas the words *usually*, *sometimes*, *often*, *seldom*, and *generally* are often found in true statements. Such words can be used as long as they don't give away the right answer.

Finally, be sure to alter the positions of the correct answers in a series of multiple-choice questions. Students soon discover that a teacher tends to make *b* or *c* the correct answer on most items. The letters should be correct answers in approximately equal numbers and should be varied in placement so that the same letter does not appear more than two or three times in a row.

Essay questions   Although short-answer questions and essays are valuable measurement tools, they are seldom used in nursing courses. They are time consuming for students to answer, thus limiting the amount of knowledge sampling you can accomplish in an examination period. They are also difficult and time consuming to grade. On the other hand, essays lend themselves to testing the highest levels of knowing, especially analysis, synthesis, and evaluation. They sometimes need to be used when there is no other adequate way to assess the students' abilities to solve problems or synthesize knowledge.

Short-answer questions, sometimes termed *restricted response* items, place limitations on the type of response requested (Gronlund, 1976). For example:

> Explain in a few sentences why patients with lymphoma are susceptible to infection.
>
> Describe three major pathological processes involved in multiple myeloma.
>
> List two infection prevention measures a nurse should teach a patient who is going home with an ileal conduit.

Full essay questions are relatively unrestricted and permit the test taker to select all pertinent information, organize it as desired, and express it in a clear manner. Here is an example of an unrestricted essay question:

> Compare two theories of death and dying, and describe how the nurse's role in supporting a dying patient might differ depending on which of the theories the nurse subscribes to.

When grading short-answer and essay questions, the teacher should have an outline of both information that must appear in the answer and information that would be desirable. Full essays can also be graded according to how well the content is organized or expressed or whether it is grammatically correct, although these types of evaluation are probably more appropriate for term papers than for examination questions.

Test Item Analysis   After a test has been constructed, given, and graded, one step still remains: performing an item analysis on objective items that provides data about the worth of the items—specifically, their level of difficulty and ability to discriminate between students who know the material and those who don't. It is useful to calculate the degree of item difficulty because very easy or very difficult questions serve little purpose. Teachers generally try to write questions that 50%–75% of the students get correct. Item difficulty is calculated by dividing the number of people who got the item right by the total number of people in the sample. The resulting percentage provides an estimate of difficulty, with the higher percentages indicating easier questions.

Item discrimination is an estimate of the usefulness of an item in differentiating between students who did well on the whole test and those who performed poorly (Hills, 1981). In other words, a discriminating question is one that the students who did well on the rest of the test got right but students who didn't do well on the test got wrong. The process for calculating item discrimination involves ranking the test papers from highest to lowest scores and choosing the top 25%–30% and the bottom 25%–30%. If you had 50 test papers, you would select the top 13–15 papers and the bottom 13–15 papers. If papers 13 and 14 both had the same grade, you would include both in the sample. Next, for each group and each test question, you would tabulate the number of people who selected each option. Your final tally for a multiple-choice question might look like this:

	Question 1			
Papers	a	b	c	d
Highest 13	1	3	9	0
Lowest 13	3	5	2	3

In looking at this chart, you can see that 9 of the 13 test takers in the highest group got the item correct (answer *c*), while only 2 of the 13 in the lowest group got it right. Obviously, the item is discriminating.

   You can do one more calculation to arrive at a *discrimination index* (Gronlund, 1976). Subtract the number of people in the lowest group who got the item right (*RL*) from the number in the highest group who got it right (*RH*) and divide by half of the sample size ($^1/_2N$). The formula appears like this:

$$D = \frac{RH - RL}{^1/_2N}$$

In the case of our hypothetical test:

$$D = \frac{9-2}{13} = .54$$

This number is an average discrimination index. All questions with a positive discrimination index are potentially useful. The best discrimination index is 1.0 and the worst is a negative number. A negative number indicates that more people in the highest group got the question wrong than those in the lowest group. Such questions are flawed in either content or format and should be discarded from the test and reworked before being used again. Likewise, questions that turn out to be too easy or too difficult should be adjusted before being used again.

An item analysis thus serves two purposes. It helps the teacher give more valid grades on the exam being analyzed, and it enables him or her to build a file of well-constructed test items for future use. In many institutions, teachers have access to computer programs that can run extensive item analyses, which can save a lot of teacher time.

It should be obvious by now that test writing is a time-consuming task that warrants a lot of attention. Because so much hinges on grades, instructors must be careful to ensure that these grades are a fair and true indication of student learning. No matter how good a teacher one is, one's reputation with students can be tainted by administering poorly developed or unfair tests. Test construction is a skill that can be learned and must be learned well.

Conducting the Class

The planning is done. You are prepared to enter the classroom the the first day of a course. What is the best way to proceed so that the class gets off to a good start, with an optimal atmosphere for learning? Let's explore some of the ways that you can make each class as positive and productive an experience as possible, for both you and the students.

The First Class: Setting the Tone and Communicating Expectations

The way you approach the first session often sets the atmosphere for the whole semester. Unless you already know every student in the class, begin by introducing yourself. In fact, to avoid future embarrassment, write your name on the board. In my early teaching days I assumed that if a student registered for my course, he or she would automatically know my name from the registration forms or booklets. It was a humbling experience to discover that some students couldn't care less who was teaching the course and had no idea who I was or how to address me. If you have a definite preference for a form of address, such as first name, "Professor," "Doctor," "Mrs.," "Sir," or whatever, make it known at the outset.

You can establish a pleasant atmosphere by welcoming the class, reading names and getting the correct pronunciations, making sure that everyone gets the handouts, and commiserating with students over the prices of textbooks, the early or late hour of the class, or the difficulty of getting back to the routine after a vacation. A little humor is helpful on the first day if it flows naturally. You can communicate an interest in students and a desire to help them by informing them of your office hours and your office phone number, thereby letting them know that you are accessible to them.

The first session is also the best time to communicate your expectations for the course. Review the course syllabus (do not, however, read it aloud word for word), and take time to answer questions about content, methods, assignments, and grading. Although you may not go through each assignment in great detail, you should at least give a general idea of the work requirements so that students can plan out their workload for the semester.

Besides content expectations, you should cover general classroom rules. If you have rules or policies about attendance and lateness, let everyone know right away and indicate the penalties for breaking the rules. It is poor practice to let the students think they can do what they like about attending class while you continue to get more and more annoyed until you end up blowing your top about students not coming to class or coming in late. Likewise, if you have rules about coming to class prepared, about tape-recording lectures, or about bringing food to class, announce them on the first day so that everyone will know your expectations.

A positive way to end this introductory portion of the course is to try to whet the students' appetites for what is to come. Try to place the course into a larger perspective for the students. Talk about why they should take this course (even if it is required), how it will help them, how they will be able to apply it to their lives, what they will like about it. If you can communicate your enthusiasm for the subject by the end of the first class, you may have given the students something to look forward to for the rest of the semester.

Subsequent Classes

In each following class, it is important to begin by gaining and controlling the attention of the students. You can easily get the attention of some groups with just a look; others practically need a police whistle. But gain their attention you must before you start to teach. If you begin talking while the group is still moving around and conversing, not only will they miss what you say but you will establish an impression of lack of control. It sometimes helps to walk around the periphery of the desks instead of standing behind the teacher's desk or lectern. Your close proximity may help establish your presence and authority. When you are close to the students, it is also easier for them to hear you as you ask them to settle down. Many teachers have also found it helpful to move about the room periodically throughout the class time and to sometimes stand in front of the teacher's desk rather than behind it to help relax the atmosphere.

As you begin the work of the course, you will need to assess the students to determine their backgrounds and how much they already know about the content of the course. This assessment can be done formally by giving pretests or short questionnaires or more informally by asking questions during class. It is equally as harmful to assume that the students already know a lot about the subject as to assume that they know nothing. If they indeed know little about the subject, you will cause great confusion by beginning to teach above the introductory level, but if they already know the material you're covering, boredom may set in.

Assessing comprehension of your teaching is also essential. Take your cues from the expressions on students' faces and from their body language, as well as from their questions. Are they understanding what you are teaching? If not, maybe you need to go over it again, explain it in a different way, or give a few examples. If no one is asking questions, ask some yourself to assess comprehension. Don't wait until the written exam to find out that the students didn't grasp what you were teaching. If possible, spend a few minutes at the end of class summarizing what you have covered and telling the students how you expect them to prepare for the next class.

Considering Students as Individuals

Earlier in this chapter, I talked about the necessity of assessing classes as groups: finding out what they know and don't know, how motivated they are, what they are like. This group approach has been the focus of most educators over the years. But recently, researchers have provided a great deal of evidence about individual learning styles in the classroom, and it seems that it may no longer be sufficient to focus on the needs of the class in general; we may have to turn our attention to the needs of individual students.

If we ignore information about students' learning-style preferences and cognitive styles, we may be bypassing an avenue for ensuring that each student will learn as much as possible.

Unfortunately, application of the research and theory of individual learning styles is scant. Many books and articles have been written about individuality in learning, but relatively little has been put into practice. Also lacking are demonstration projects and evaluative research that would help teachers place confidence in the practicality and value of attending to individual learning styles. So, I will simply present an overview of the information that is available, give some suggestions for how teachers might use this information, point out some of the problems involved in applying this body of knowledge, and leave it up to you to judge the worth and usefulness of an individualized approach to teaching and learning.

Three aspects of the study of individual learning styles have emerged over the last 25 years: students' learning-style preferences, students' cognitive style, and students' response style. Learning-style preference is probably the only aspect that has been applied in nursing education.

Learning-Style Preferences

Researchers who have investigated *learning-style preferences* usually base their work on the premise that students develop preferred ways of learning because of such things as their personality, intelligence, biological rhythms, personal goals, or learning environment. People differ in their preferences for learning atmospheres, classroom structures, types of teachers, and modes of teaching. Students may feel more comfortable when learning a certain preferred way and may learn more or more effectively when using the preferred style, although research has yet to fully substantiate this (Ostmoe et al, 1984).

Several models have been proposed to explain learning-style preferences, and several instruments have been developed to diagnose these preferences. Kolb developed a model of experiential learning and a learning-style inventory for young adults based on four preferred ways of learning: (1) *concrete experience* (becoming actively involved in a situation), (2) *reflective observation* (observing and thinking about experiences), (3) *abstract conceptualization* (deriving concepts and theories from observation), and (4) *active experimentation* (testing hypotheses and problem solving). Although learners may, and ideally should, use all these modes of learning,

Kolb suggests that learners have preferences for specific modes (Dunn et al, 1981).

Canfield's model of learning style applies to junior high school through adult levels (Merritt, 1983). He proposed that learners have preferences for the conditions under which learning takes place and for the sensory modes of learning. The conditions he delineated are (1) *affiliation* (friendly relationships with instructors and peers), (2) *structure* (desire for organization and detail), (3) *achievement* (freedom to set goals and study independently), and (4) *eminence* (desire for competition and learning from an authority on a subject). The sensory preferences he defined are (1) *listening*, (2) *reading*, (3) *iconics* (visual, media), and (4) *direct experience*. Canfield also developed an instrument to assess these learning styles.

A number of other models and assessment tools have been published. Many have been developed by researchers devising new instruments and models for their own work, and all are based on some aspect of learning theory. The following research is indicative of the use of some of these models.

In 1974, Canfield and Lafferty (using an earlier version of the Canfield instrument just described) compared preferred learning styles of students studying criminal justice, preeducation, physical therapy, nursing, and Girl Scout administration (cited in Payton et al, 1979). Criminal justice and preeducation students rated high on the need for competition and authority. Physical therapy and baccalaureate nursing students expressed strong needs for organization and direct experience. The researchers also found differences between male and female students, with women having a greater preference for organization and people-directed content and men preferring numeric and inanimate content.

Rezler and French (1975) devised a Learning Preferences Inventory, which they used to measure learning preferences of students in six allied health professions. Their inventory encompassed six dimensions: (1) *abstract* (preference for learning theories, principles, and concepts), (2) *concrete* (preference for learning practical skills), (3) *individual* (preference for working alone), (4) *interpersonal* (preference for working in harmonious relationships with others), (5) *student-structured* (preference for autonomy and self-direction), and (6) *teacher-structured* (preference for learning in an organized, teacher-directed class). The researchers found few differences among the six health profession groups, but they did note pronounced preferences for learning styles within the professional groups. For example, "the majority of students in all six groups preferred concrete tasks assigned by the teacher" (p. 23). However, there were students in most groups who preferred abstract learning and self-structured learning.

A study of learning style preferences of ADN students was conducted by Ferrell in 1978. The subjects were LPNs or the equivalent who were entering a one-year associate degree nursing program in which the objectives were to be met through modules of mostly independent learning. Those responsible for the program wanted to be sure that the modules would enable students to use their own learning style and that the students were reasonably self-directed. Two instruments were used. The first, a Learning Styles Inventory developed by Renzulli and Smith in 1974, was designed to assess how students felt about nine learning methods: projects, simulation, drill and recitation, peer teaching, discussion, games, independent study, programmed instruction, and lecture (cited in Ferrell, 1978). The second instrument was an attitude scale developed by the researchers to determine how autonomous students were in their attitudes toward learning. Only composite scores were reported. All of the learning methods were found to be acceptable to the subjects, with the exception of simulation. The method most highly rated was peer teaching. The students as a group tended to be autonomous learners; they reported that the modules enabled them to use the learning styles they preferred.

In 1979 Payton, Hueter, and McDonald reported a study of learning-style preferences of 1,099 physical therapy students. The instrument used was the Canfield and Lafferty 1974 Learning Styles Inventory. This instrument measured conditions for learning, such as the needs for affiliation, structure, achievement, and eminence. It also measured preferred content areas, encompassing such things as number, qualitative, inanimate, and people orientations, and it assessed preferred modes of learning, including listening, reading, iconics (visual), and direct experience. Results indicated that, in general, physical therapy students were neutral in their preference for working with peers, setting their own objectives, working with inanimate objects, and learning by visual illustrations. The students preferred to work closely with the instructor and other people, liked course work to be well organized, and preferred to learn by listening and direct experience. They had low interest in independent action, working alone, competing with others, working with numbers and words, and reading. Differences between men and women students were negligible. The researchers believed that the individual inventory results could be used in classroom and clinical settings to tailor learning to individual needs.

Merritt (1983) used the Kolb and Canfield models and inventories to determine whether there were differences between learning-style preferences of basic nursing students and RN students in a baccalaureate nursing program. She initially found no differences between the learning-style preferences of the two groups. However, when the mean scores were adjusted for age and work experiences, she found that basic students had a greater preference for structure, affiliation, achievement, direct experience, and iconics.

In a 1984 study, a learning strategy questionnaire was developed and administered to two groups of baccalaureate nursing students (Ostmoe et al, 1984). One group was just beginning the nursing curriculum, while the second was completing the last nursing course. Both groups preferred lecture, live demonstration, textbook, required readings, films, and case studies. The beginning students generally had more favorable attitudes toward a greater variety of strategies. The senior group had several strategies they "seldom" preferred, including television lecture, audiotapes, audiovisual self-instruction, programmed instruction, independent study, role playing, and computer-assisted instruction.

The research that has been done to apply preferred-learning-style theory is in its infancy. But some worthwhile questions and ideas for application have been raised. These implications will be discussed later.

Cognitive Style

The term *cognitive style* refers to consistent ways in which individuals organize and process information from their environment. It includes their ways of thinking, perceiving, and remembering. As with preferred learning style, there are quite a few models of cognitive style and accompanying instruments to measure the traits identified. All of these models have implications for individual learning styles in the classroom.

The best-known and most studied cognitive-style model is Witkin's *field independence–field dependence* model. Witkin (and others following him) has described a bipolar continuum of ways in which people approach their environment, from analytically to globally (Messick, 1976). A strongly field-independent person perceives figures as discernible from their backgrounds and easily perceives objects and ideas that are embedded in a context. A strongly field-dependent person has a more global approach and tends to perceive total configurations rather than separate parts. Field-independent persons have been found to be more adept at task analysis, problem solving, and cognitive pursuits than field-dependent people. They are more individualistic, more aloof, and less effective at social skills. Conversely, field-dependent people are sociable, have a concern for people, and are better at learning material with social content and at conflict resolution.

Three classic tests or tasks are used to determine a person's degree of field independence/dependence: the Rod and Frame test, the Body Adjustment test, and the Embedded Figures test. They can be used separately or in combination to assess students for their position on the continuum.

A second cognitive-style model is Ragan's distinction between *reflection* and *impulsivity*. This model describes the differences in how people respond to a confronting problem. Reflective individuals tend to spend time thinking about and evaluating alternative hypotheses and solutions, whereas impulsive individuals select or try the first solution that occurs to them and are often wrong. The most commonly used test of reflection-impulsivity is the Matching Familiar Figures test (Ragan et al, 1979).

Integrative complexity is a third way of looking at cognitive style. The promise of this model is that people process information in two ways: differentiation and integration. *Differentiation* refers to an individual's ability to separate incoming stimuli into dimensions (for example, perceiving the three dimensions of color as hue, brightness, and saturation). *Integration* is the person's ability to combine the dimensions into a complex schema. A person who rates low in differentiating and integrating ability is called *concrete*, while the person who rates highly on these cognitive tasks is termed *abstract*. A concrete individual is one who tends to put thoughts and beliefs into compartments, to see things as black or white, and to generalize a great deal. He or she may place great reliance on authority, may be unable to see alternative solutions to problems, and may not handle stress well. The abstract person can process large amounts of complex information, functions well in unstructured environments, and handles stress well. Several tools can be used to measure integrative complexity, including the This I Believe test, the Sentence Completion test, and the Paragraph Completion test (Goldstein & Blackman, 1987).

A number of other, lesser known cognitive-style models relate to some aspect of the way people deal with incoming stimuli. All have implications for how students learn and how instructors teach.

Response Style

Another aspect of learning style is the way in which students behave and interact in the classroom, a field of study called *student response style*. Both educators and psychologists have done research in this area and have developed some models.

The Mann model evolved from a study of 96 college students who were interviewed and observed. This study revealed that students fell into eight response types: compliant students, anxious-dependent students, discouraged workers, independent students, heroes, snipers, attention seekers, and silent students. Half of the students clustered into the categories of anxious-dependent and silent students, all of whom had low self-evaluations and had feelings of helplessness (Partridge, 1983).

The *Grasha-Riechmann* model was also developed as a result of studying college students (Riechmann & Grasha, 1974). Six response styles (three bipolar continuums) emerged: independent, dependent, participant, avoidant, collaborative, and competitive. The researchers developed the Grasha-Riechmann Student Learning Style Scales to measure student response types. Although there are other models, you can get an idea of the realm of response types from these examples, and you can probably recognize some of these types even without testing your students.

Implications for Teaching

A wealth of information is available in the learning-style literature that can help teachers scientifically individualize student learning. The question is whether educators are willing to change their thinking and their methods and do the extra work that it takes to design individual learning.

One hurdle that has to be taken before instructional designs can be formulated is testing students to determine their learning styles. How often should students be tested, using which tests, and how many of them? Should students be tested in each course, in each department, or by the parent institution on admission? How should student learning styles be communicated to teachers (if they are not assessed by each teacher)?

After assessment of learning styles, further questions arise. Should students always be matched with their preferred instructional mode or cognitive style? Isn't there a danger of helping students to become too rigid, unable to learn comfortably with a new structure if that is necessary? Should educators purposefully try to build up students' weak areas in learning style so that they can benefit from universal approaches? Would a commitment to individualization in teaching mean that each student would have a series of optional approaches? Chapter 6 provides more insight into the ways that individualized learning can be structured.

One practical application of learning-style theory is that once educators know a student's learning style (preferred modes, cognitive and response styles), they can use that information in student counseling and tutoring. If a student has problems with study skills, he or she can be directed to study methods most suited to his or her style. Tutors can also use methods that are most likely to help individual students learn.

Further research into the effectiveness of matching students with instructional modes will give greater credence to the applicability and value of this approach. As evidence begins to build in the case for individuality in learning, more teachers may be won over to it.

References

Bloom BS: *Taxonomy of Educational Objectives.* Longman, 1984.

Brown JW, Lewis RB, Harcleroad FF: *AV Instruction: Media and Methods* 3d ed. McGraw-Hill, 1969.

Carlson SB: *Creative Classroom Testing.* Educational Testing Service, 1985.

Dunn R et al: Learning style researchers define differences differently. *Educ Leadership* 1981; 38:372–375.

Eble KE: *The Craft of Teaching.* Jossey-Bass, 1976.

Ferrell B: Attitudes toward learning styles and self-direction of ADN students. *J Nurs Educ* (Feb) 1978; 17:19–22.

Gage NL (editor): *The Psychology of Teaching Methods.* U Chicago Press, 1976.

Gallo BM, Gallo DR: Guided reading: a strategy to enhance learning. *J Nurs Educ* (Jan) 1974; 13:21–25.

Goldstein KM, Blackman S: *Cognitive Style: Five Approaches and Relevant Research.* Wiley, 1978.

Gronlund NE: *Measurement and Evaluation in Teaching* 3d ed. Macmillan, 1976.

Hills JR: *Measurement and Evaluation in the Classroom* 2d ed. Merrill, 1981.

McKeachie WJ: *Teaching Tips: A Guidebook for the Beginning College Teacher.* Heath, 1969.

Merritt SL: Learning style preferences of baccalaureate nursing students. *Nurs Res* 1983; 32:367–372.

Messick S: *Individuality in Learning.* Jossey-Bass, 1976.

Ostmoe PM et al: Learning style preferences and selection of learning strategies: consideration and implications for nurse educators. *J Nurs Educ* (Jan) 1984; 23:27–30.

Parsons M, O'Shea HS: Textbook selection: perils and pointers. *J Nurs Educ* 1986; 25:343–345.

Partridge R: Learning styles: a review of selected models. *J Nurs Educ* 1983; 22:243–248.

Payton OD, Hueter AE, McDonald ME: Learning style preferences. *Physical Therapy* 1979; 59:147–152.

Ragan TJ et al: *Cognitive Styles: a Review of the Literature.* Air Force Systems Command, 1979.

Rezler AG, French RM: Personality types and learning preferences of students in six allied health professions. *J Allied Health* 1975; 4:20–26.

Riechmann SW, Grasha AF: A rational approach to developing and assessing the construct validity of a student learning style scales instrument. *J Psych* 1974; 87(1st half):213–223.

Ryan TA: Research: guide for teaching improvement. *Improving College and University Teaching* 1968; 17:270–276.

PART

II

TEACHING
METHODS

Chapter 4

Lecture, Discussion, Questioning

The lecture method of teaching has been around longer than any other and is used most often, but in recent decades it has suffered a rather negative image. However, people often refer to different things when they use the word *lecture*. To some it means the formal lectures that have been around since the Middle Ages, in which the lecturer does all the talking from a prepared script and perhaps allows time for questions at the end. To others it means a combination of lecturing, discussion between students and lecturer, and questioning by the teacher. Still others include the use of audiovisuals or props within the context of a lecture.

The first part of this chapter discusses the lecture in its traditional sense, of information being conveyed verbally and quite formally by the lecturer with little teacher-student interaction; this method is still widely used today. Then the topics of discussion and questioning are explored, with an explanation of how they are often woven together in the modern form of the lecture that I call the interactive lecture.

Formal Lectures

When lectures were used in the Middle Ages, they were a method of conveying facts, information, and ideas that could not readily be obtained elsewhere. Books, charts, and tapes were not available, so the lecture became a necessary means of teaching. Today we have so many ways of conveying information that it is often argued that we no longer need the lecture method. Opponents claim that lectures force students into a passive role. They believe that students could learn the same information more efficiently by reading and that most teachers lecture simply because it is the way that they were taught. Proponents of the lecture method such as Hyman (1974) believe that the faults are in the users, not in the method, and that lecturing can serve many educational purposes.

Purposes of Lectures

Lectures can be an efficient means for introducing students to new topics. Once the teacher has used lecture to set the stage for a new area of learning and has put the new field into the perspective of what is already known, he or she might use other methods to teach the body of material. For example, an instructor might use a formal lecture to introduce the topic of fluid/electrolyte balance and relate it to what students know about homeostasis and nourishment. He or she could then use other strategies to develop the topic further.

Another purpose of the lecture method is to integrate and synthesize knowledge from several fields or sources. Synthesis can be done more readily by a knowledgeable teacher than by a student who is a novice in the field. Take the topic of quality assurance, for example. A teacher can use lecture to elucidate the models of quality assurance and the many ways that they can be applied in the health care field. It would take a learner an inordinate amount of time to pull together all of this information about quality assurance and to make sense of it all.

The lecture method can also be used to arouse students' interest in a subject. Reading about pharmacology may be a sure way to make the uninitiated student believe that it's a dull subject indeed. However, an enlivening introductory lecture on pharmacology would enable the student to see it as a fascinating subject that just might be interesting to study.

Difficult concepts can be clarified in lectures. Concepts such as arrhythmia, compensation in acid-base balance, or increased intra-cranial pressure may be explained best by the lecture method, especially with the added use of the blackboard to help graphically portray the concepts. Other methods are often not as effective in bringing order to the students' thinking on such subjects.

Lectures can serve as a means of preparing for a discussion. Students have to have something concrete to discuss, and although they often prepare by reading, the topics are sometimes better introduced by lecture to set the stage for fruitful and pointed discussions

Finally, the lecture format can be used to analyze a problem or theory. The teacher can verbally demonstrate the problem-solving process and show the students how a learned person goes about solving a problem or analyzing a theory or a clinical situation. Other specific applications of the lecture method undoubtedly exist as well. The success of the lecture in fulfilling its purposes often depends, however, on the techniques used by the lecturer.

Lecturing Techniques

Many educators extol the proper techniques of lecturing, but in actual practice such techniques are not used on a consistent basis. Teachers need to learn the techniques and review them once in a while to prevent their lectures from falling into undesirable ruts. It is helpful to remember, though, that even the best lecturers sometimes give bad lectures. When teachers give a lecture that they know has not been good (and they are usually aware of it), they can use the experience to learn about the pitfalls of lecturing and try to avoid them in the future.

Following are techniques that can aid in delivering interesting, lively, and even memorable lectures. Keep in mind, however, that the content of the lecture is more important than technique, and all of the lecturing techniques in the world cannot make a good lecture out of poorly conceived content. Once you have selected and organized your information (as discussed in Chapter 3), you can focus your attention on technique.

Spontaneity   The most valuable piece of advice I can give about lecture technique is to avoid reading to the class. Reading kills all spontaneity and can be anesthetizing. To avoid the temptation to read (and it is a great temptation if you are anxious), do not write your lecture out in full sentences. If your notes are in the form of lists and phrases, you will have to think during the delivery and spontaneity will increase. If you review your notes before the lecture, and in the beginning try rehearsing the delivery at home, you will feel secure enough without a written script in front of you. I would not recommend trying to do without any notes. Organization of the lecture could suffer if you forget the order in which you planned your content. It is also possible for any lecturer to draw a blank for a moment and be unable to recall what comes next—notes are a lifesaver in such instances.

Voice Quality   If your voice is not loud enough for all students to hear easily, use a microphone if possible. When I first began teaching, my voice was tight because of my anxiety, and I could not project it well. It wasn't until I read the students' evaluations at the end of the course that I realized how frustrating it was for them to have to strain to hear me.

In addition to volume, beware of lecturing in a monotone. Anxiety and boredom with the content can lead to monotone delivery. It takes some practice to periodically alter both pitch and volume while lecturing. If you are enthusiastic about your topic, your voice can show it. Palmer (1983) goes so far as to recommend studying the performing arts if you need to in order to control your voice, improve your speaking ability, and make your lectures more dramatic.

Body Language   You can also add to the dramatic quality of your lecturing by your movements. Do not stand glued to one spot in back of a podium, hanging on to it for security. Move a little to one side occasionally, or move in front of the lectern or podium to bring yourself in closer contact with the students. Use your hands for emphasis, but don't wave them around so much that they are distracting. Be aware of your body language. Constantly keeping your arms crossed or keeping your hands clasped behind your back can connote anxiety. Maintain eye contact with the audience as much as possible. Avoid looking out the window, at the wall, or above the students' heads, all of which give the impression that you are afraid of or uninvolved with the class.

If you have ever been in a class with a teacher who has annoying mannerisms, you know how distracting they can be. The types of mannerisms that teachers display are legion. Some are habits of movement, such as pacing, clicking fingers, bending a paperclip, tossing chalk, jingling coins in a pocket, pushing eyeglasses up, or using two fingers to represent quotation marks. Verbal habits may be even worse, such as frequently saying "uh," "er," "okay?" or "and so forth." Such patterns are easy to fall into and hard to break; in fact, lecturers are often unaware of them unless someone points them out. Watching yourself on a videotape or even listening to your lecture on audiotape can be useful in helping you to see yourself as others see you, mannerisms and all.

Pacing   The pacing of a lecture affects the students' comprehension and enjoyment of the material. Too slow a pace can induce boredom, but too fast a pace can cause writer's cramp as students struggle to take notes; students need to have some time to interpret what the teacher is saying and to formulate questions. Alternating the pace makes for a more stimulating lecture. A good policy is to speak faster when covering familiar ground but pause at times to allow difficult or controversial points to sink in.

Clarification   Clarifying confusing or difficult concepts during a lecture is essential. Clarification can be done by means of structure, examples, and analogies. When Davis (1965) observed master lecturers, he found two commonalities among them. First, lecture plans were simple. The content was not simplistic, but the lecture was built around a simple plan, such as four kinds of economic markets or five steps in the decision-making process. A nursing lecture might be built around the illness experience and the recovery process, the five steps of the nursing process, or three models of client teaching. If the plan is simple and is made evident to the students, it can help them organize and remember information more effectively.

   The second quality that Davis noted about popular master lecturers was their abundant use of examples. Whether from real life or hypothetical, examples not only clarify but also help apply concepts. For instance, in a lecture about research hypotheses, a score of examples from actual research could be used to explain and apply the need for hypotheses, how they are developed, and the types that exist.

   Analogies can also be used for clarification. Likening an atherosclerotic vessel to a blocked drain pipe, or relating the immune reaction to the mobilization of an army, can help students move more easily from the known to the unknown.

Visual Aids   A formal lecture need not employ only the spoken word. The blackboard, charts, graphs, and other visual materials can be used for illustration. These aids can also help with clarification and retention of information. Referring to a chart or picture can be invaluable in fixing information in a student's memory, while placing the outline of the lecture plan on the blackboard emphasizes the key points of the lecture.

Key Points   A good lecture focuses on just a few important points, which it expands and exemplifies. When preparing your notes and reviewing them before class, think about the three or four things you would most like the students to remember from this lecture 6 months or a year later. If, for example, you are giving a lecture on increased intracranial pressure, you might want the students to remember the early warning signs, pathologic results of increased pressure, and nursing measures to reduce the pressure.

Even if you are covering other material in your lecture, the three main aspects will be the ones that you thoroughly explain and that you emphasize by voice, gestures, and visual effects. You can also add emphasis by providing examples from real clients in your practice or from hypothetical client situations. It is not enough to highlight these three important areas in your objectives; you must emphasize them during the lecture.

Another means of fixing important concepts in the students' minds is summarizing at transitional points in the lecture or at the end. Repetition in the form of summaries will highlight important features and help the students put all of the information into perspective.

Question Periods   Finally, a technique that should always be used, even in a formal lecture, is allowing time for questions. If the lecture has transitional points, as when moving from the topic of incipient increased intracranial pressure to the management of acute pressure, you might plan time for questions then. If questions during the lecture would be disruptive, allow time at the end. Rather than asking, "Are there any questions?" be a little more specific and ask, "Are there any questions relating to _____ or _____?" Soliciting participation in this way encourages people to narrow their thoughts to specific areas. It is also helpful to repeat each person's question so that everyone in the room can hear it; it is disturbing to hear supposedly informative answers to questions one hasn't heard. Repeating the question also gives you a chance to rephrase it for clarity if needed.

If reading about these techniques makes you realize that you need to improve your lectures, as do most teachers, my last piece of advice is to try improving one area at a time. It's not easy to change behavior, especially if habits are well entrenched. Trying to change several aspects at one time will probably end in failure. Even if you are new to teaching and don't have hardened habits, don't try to implement all of these techniques the first week. Good lecturers develop—they don't spring into the teaching world fully perfected.

Advantages of the Lecture Method

The greatest advantage of the lecture method over other methods is that it is economical. The size of the class is limited only by the classroom space. Formal lectures are just as effective for 200 students as they are for 20 as long as the lecturer has a microphone.

Lectures are also economical in terms of student time. A great deal of information can be communicated in a 1-hour lecture— usually more information than could be gained from a discussion, for instance. More pertinent information can often be taught in 1 hour than a student could learn from a textbook in that time, because the lecturer can sift through the textbook information and pull out what is most important as well as include information from other sources that it might take a student hours to locate and read.

The lecturer can supplement a textbook by enhancing a topic and making it come to life. No matter how well written, words on a page are dry and impersonal compared to words communicated by a lecturer with a wealth of personal experience and enthusiasm for the subject. A good lecturer can inspire an audience in a way that few textbooks can.

During a lecture, a teacher serves as a role model for students. He or she actively demonstrates the thinking processes of a scholar and serves as an example of an expert in the field as well as a good public speaker. Students need to see this kind of role modeling.

Opponents of the lecture method argue that lecturing causes students to be in a passive role, but that is not necessarily true. A well-designed and well-delivered lecture can stimulate students' minds and keep them alert and questioning, pondering the problems and issues raised in the lecture. As Heller states, "To equate physical passivity with mental inactivity is to admit ignorance of logic, semantics, and psychology" (1962; 100). Physical activity and verbal exchanges between teacher and student are not necessary for active learning to take place.

An advantage of the one-way verbal communication is that it helps students develop their listening abilities. Nurses need to be good listeners on the job, so why not practice on lecturers? Listening to a lecture and trying to extract important points for note taking is good practice for listening to patients and making mental or written notes of what they say.

Lectures, although they may not meet the learning needs of each individual student, can be adapted to meet the needs of the specific class group. For example, a lecture to a group of RN upper-division students could take advantage of their previous knowl-edge and interests, whereas a lecture on the same topic to generic baccalaureate students would need to be more basic.

Finally, an advantage revealed by many research studies is that students often prefer lectures over other teaching methods. Some educators attribute this preference to the fact that students don't have to work as hard as with some other methods. Although that may be part of the reason, it does not totally explain the preference for lectures. Some students like lectures because they like the large group sessions for the social contacts they make; some like them because they can gain a lot of information in a short time; and some prefer to learn from the lips of an authority and want the personal touch that comes from a teacher in the classroom rather than a videotape or a book.

The lecture method has enough advantages to support its con-tinued use. Teachers should be sure, however, that they are lectur-ing because it serves a good purpose and because it is a suitable method for the situation and not just because they don't want to take the time to think about whether another method would be better.

Disadvantages of the Lecture Method

As already mentioned, many people object to the lecture method because it places students in the passive role of a sponge, just there to soak up knowledge. Because it does not require active participa-tion from students, there is no guarantee that the objectives of the lecture are being achieved. All of this may be true if the lecture is not planned and carried out well. Even if a student is mentally active, nothing can ensure that such activity will continue for the whole lecture, and research that I describe later in the chapter points out that students rarely attend to the whole lecture.

Educators who decry the lecture method claim that few teach-ers are good lecturers and therefore few can achieve class objec-tives by this method, much less hold students' attention or serve as good role models. Because so many students are subjected to poor lectures throughout their college days, those who go on to become educators themselves often fall into the same bad habits.

The passive student role also reinforces submission to author-ity, according to Gotesky (1966). He believes that because examina-tions are often based on lecture content, students are compelled to absorb the opinions, assumptions, and even mistakes of the teacher. Thus, students are not questioning, challenging, and probing as they should but are forced to accept what is said and to repeat it back on tests.

One of the great disadvantages of the lecture method is that by nature it lends itself to the teaching of facts and information while placing little emphasis on problem solving, decision making, analytical thinking, or transfer of learning. That doesn't mean that these latter types of learning cannot take place in a lecture, but they are less likely to occur than when other methods are used.

Another serious drawback is that lecturing is not conducive to meeting students' individual learning needs. Students are limited to learning from an authority figure and learning by the stimulation of only one of the senses, hearing. In a formal lecture students have no opportunity to learn from peers, to learn by manipulation of data, to discover, to learn visually or through touch, and so on. The impersonality of large lecture classes adds to this problem of lack of individualization.

It should be clear by this point that the disadvantages to the lecture method can be minimized by not using it to the exclusion of all other teaching methods. By using a variety of strategies, the teacher can enhance the advantages of all of the techniques.

Research on Lecturing

Most of the research studies involving the lecture method are experiments in which a newer method like independent study or computer-assisted instruction is compared to lecturing on an outcome variable such as an end-of-course achievement test. Such experiments reveal more about the newer teaching method than they do about lecturing, so I have discussed them in the chapters that deal with those other methods, such as computer-assisted instruction.

Relatively little research has been done on the lecture method itself. Much of it was done 15 or 20 years ago, though the findings are still pertinent today. These studies focus mostly on measuring attention during a lecture and retention of information afterward.

In 1968 Cameron used consciousness sampling to determine what students were thinking about during a lecture (cited in Schoen, 1970). He used the rather drastic method of firing a gun 20 different times during a semester of psychology lectures and asking students to record what they were thinking about in the split second before the gun went off. He found the appalling results that on the average, only 20% of students were paying attention to the lecturer, whereas 29% were thinking erotic thoughts, 20% were reminiscing about something, and the rest were pursuing thoughts about lunch, other students, religion, or things they were worried about. Obviously, we cannot assume that these findings would hold true in all classrooms, because of such variables as teacher ability, subject content, and student personalities, but they likely apply to classrooms other than just the sample.

Schoen used similar methodology in a 1970 study with two psychology lecture classes, one undergraduate and one graduate. He used a bell as the attention device; he rang it at 10 intervals during the semester and asked students to record their thoughts. He found that 62% of undergraduates' thoughts were centered on the lecture topic, as were 72% of the graduate students'. These results are more reassuring to lecturers. Schoen also assessed student attention when other teaching methods were used and discovered that students were most attentive during problem solving and least attentive during panel discussions. The ranking of methods for attentiveness was (1) problem solving, (2) movies, (3) discussion, (4) buzz session, (5) lecture, (6) student-led exercise, and (7) panel discussion.

Another interesting piece of research was done by Thomas in 1972. He performed an experiment designed to discover how the information remembered after a lecture varies with the time at which the information is given during the lecture. The sample was 108 adults from the British Armed Services who watched a 52-minute videotaped lecture on a new system of measurement units. They were pretested and posttested with a multiple-choice exam. The results indicated that the subjects recalled about 90% of the material presented during the initial few minutes, but the percentage then began to decline rapidly until at the 45-minute point less than half of the material could be recalled. Recall of information given in the last few minutes of the lecture improved dramatically. Figure 4-1 illustrates these findings.

In 1978 Stuart and Rutherford studied the attention and concentration levels of British medical students in lectures on hematology. They found that concentration rose to a peak at 15 minutes and then fell steadily until the end of the lecture. Results were fairly uniform across several classes with different lecturers and different-level students. The researchers concluded that lectures should

Figure 4-1   **Recall During Lecture**

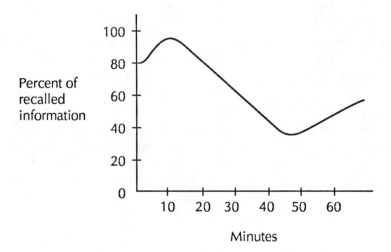

probably be shortened to 30 minutes from the conventional 50 or that a break should be given during the hour. Another approach is for the teacher to switch to another teaching method after 30 minutes.

The implication of all these studies is that lecturers need to be concerned about ways to increase student attentiveness and absorption of material, especially in the last half of the lecture.

Some of the earliest research done on the lecture method was conducted by Jones in the 1920s (cited in McLeish, 1976). This researcher conducted a series of experiments to discover ways of improving lecturing effectiveness. He came up with some interesting results. First, note taking did not make any real difference in retention of information. On the other hand, giving a quiz 5 minutes before the end of the lecture facilitated retention of the material over an 8-week period. Retention was also improved by "increasing the forcefulness, dramatic appeal, and quality of the lecture; by reducing the number of points presented and going at a slower pace; by increasing the concreteness and the number of illustrations used" (McLeish, 1976; 266).

The effectiveness of giving students written copies of a lecture has been debated over the years. In 1968 MacManaway hypothesized that giving out lecture scripts to be studied in the students' own time instead of having them attend lectures would result in more efficient note taking, would save student time, and would produce better understanding of the material. In his study, the experimental groups did not attend lectures but received the scripts; the control groups attended lectures as usual. The results indicated that private reading of lecture scripts did allow for more efficient note taking, was slightly *more* time consuming, and resulted in greater understanding of the material. Other outcomes, such as student interest and attitude change, were not measured.

McLeish (1976) conducted an experiment in which 60 architectural students were assigned to one of three groups. Group I students were asked to spend 1 hour reading a lecture script on a subject that they would soon apply in class. Group II were given the lecture orally and told that they would soon be using the information and that they should take notes and think of ways to apply the material. Group III students only heard the lecture, with no special preparation. On a written test of immediate recall, Group I scored 50%, Groups II and III 40%. A week later all three groups scored 35% on the test. McLeish concluded that "irrespective of differences due to the teaching methods used, the work which students do for themselves in preparation for an examination will tend to bring their scores close to equality" (1976; 271).

Whether students gain as much from reading a textbook as they do from lectures plus the textbook is another question that has often been asked. Marr et al (1960) studied 144 undergraduate students in an introductory psychology course to find some answers to this question. Formal lectures were given at each class meeting for the control group. The experimental group received no formal lectures but read the material in the textbook and met with a teacher once a week so that their questions on the reading could be answered. As measured by scores on subsequent multiple-choice examinations, the group that received lectures (the control group) did significantly better than the group that did not receive lectures.

The research done on the lecture method is not extensive, but the findings are interesting. More research needs to be designed to determine effective lecture methods. For example, what role does lecture formality or informality play in determining learning outcomes? Does humor enhance lectures? What are the interaction effects between teacher personality and lecture methods? Research on the effectiveness of lectures versus discussion is examined in the next section.

Discussion

The term *discussion* has many meanings. It is sometimes used syn-
onymously with *seminar, debate,* or *panel.* It may include teacher- or
student-led, formal or informal discussions. I will use the term in
the sense of formal teacher-led discussions. Debates and seminars
are separate entities and will be dealt with in Chapter 5.

Formal discussion involves an interchange of informed opinions and reactions, group consideration of a problem or issue,
sharing of ideas and information, and exchange of questions and
answers. It is structured to have both participants and a leader or
moderator and to achieve instructional objectives.

Purposes of Discussion

Discussions serve many educational purposes. The most obvious is
probably to give students an opportunity to apply principles, concepts, and theories and, in that process, to transfer their learning to
new and different situations. This approach presupposes that students have already learned a body of information on which they
will base their discussion. For example, a group of nurses may have
heard an inservice lecture on management styles or read some
articles about management theories. They may then come together
for a discussion about management as it takes place on specific
patient care units.

A related purpose is clarification of information and concepts.
Thus, the group discussing management theory may have as an
objective the clarification of concepts of management as they were
presented in the lecture and readings. While this mystifying and
obscure information is being made clear to the students (by explanations from the instructor or from other students) the teacher is
receiving feedback about the participants' grasp of the material
and the achievement of objectives. The discussion method, perhaps
more than any other, helps the teacher gauge student understanding as learning is taking place. Misconceptions and hazy thinking
can be assessed and corrected immediately.

Through discussions, students can learn the process of group
problem solving. The discussion group may be divided into subgroups so that each can work on some aspect of the problem, or the
entire group can work together toward a solution. From this interaction, students learn how different people apply the steps of the
problem-solving process, and they learn to draw on the expertise of

group members, capitalizing on each other's strengths. An example of group problem solving with beginning students might be a discussion of ways to alleviate anxiety in hospitalized people; with upper-level students, it could be a discussion of ways to improve the image of the nursing profession.

Part of the socialization of a professional is to learn the group process and how to become an effective team member. Group discussion is a valuable tool in helping students work cooperatively and collaboratively under the guidance of a faculty member. Students can learn to value the contributions of others and to develop team spirit.

Discussions about professional, societal, or ethical issues can help students develop and evaluate their beliefs and positions. In the give and take with other group members, they learn whether their position is clear, logical, and defensible. They get immediate feedback on the position they have taken. At the same time, they are listening to the arguments of others, analyzing and weighing them, accepting or rejecting them. In other words, students are getting practice in using critical thinking skills. A corollary to this purpose is that discussion helps students sharpen their ability to express themselves. With practice, they realize what they have to say and how they have to say it if they are to make their point and have an impact on the group.

Attitudes can be changed through discussion. As students hear other viewpoints and begin to look at issues and situations through the eyes and experiences of others, their own attitudes can change. Students also learn that it is possible to change the attitudes of others through group discussion.

Discussions can raise students' interest and enthusiasm for a subject or a course and can therefore increase their motivation to attend class and to learn. A substantial amount of research supports students' preference for discussions over many other teaching methods.

Discussion Techniques

Good discussions do not just happen spontaneously; they require careful planning. The teacher must develop objectives and choose appropriate topics. Not all class material lends itself to the formal discussion method. For example, it would be difficult to hold a lively discussion about the immune response. Topics that are most suitable for discussion are controversial issues, clinical or professional problems, and emotionally laden topics such as death and dying. It is possible to have discussions about factual material like the pathophysiology of toxemia, but what would be gained by taking the time to discuss facts when they could be read or lectured on more efficiently? A discussion of factual material that students are having difficulty understanding may be appropriate. The teacher can simplify and clarify the information and then help the students apply it.

After choosing a topic, the instructor is responsible for providing some structure for the discussion. The teacher should make sure that students know how they are to prepare for the class. He or she may want them to read a chapter in the textbook, read some articles, or recall some personal experience that would be pertinent. Building a discussion around a common experience is often worthwhile. The teacher may ask the students to attend a professional program or watch a television show, or he or she may show a film at the beginning of class as a taking-off point for the discussion. The teacher then directs the course of the discussion so that the objectives are met. This can be done by writing the objectives on the blackboard or by introducing topics and questions periodically so that all necessary aspects are covered.

In addition to structuring the content, the teacher or group should set some ground rules. These rules may include time limits for various aspects of the discussion, prohibitions against interrupting someone, or limits on the number of times any one person may speak.

Planning of a discussion should also take the physical environment into consideration. Ideally, the classroom will permit chairs to be arranged so that everyone can sit in a circle. The more eye contact among participants, the better the possibilities for a good discussion. Forming a circle also makes it easier for all to hear. If a large class must be broken into several small discussion groups, the room should be large enough to allow space between groups. The teacher will then have to move around from group to group, monitoring their progress.

Once the discussion is under way, the teacher takes on the role of facilitator and leader. This role entails several functions. First, the leader should refrain from doing much talking. That isn't easy when the teacher is used to being the information source and resident expert in the classroom, but his or her entering into the discussion, however valuable the information offered, serves only to intimidate the students and decrease their participation. Rather than participating, the leader's role is to encourage others to participate.

Encouraging quiet members of the group to contribute is a challenge. It helps to make eye contact with them and smile. The teacher may direct simple questions to them or draw on their personal experiences or expertise. The instructor might say, "Debbie, what do you think about what Jane has just said in light of your experience with Mrs. S. in the clinical area last week?" Although it is important to encourage reticent students, it should not always be mandatory that every student talk. Beginning students may need time to adjust to college life and group work and may adjust best if allowed the freedom simply to listen. When quiet students do participate, they should be rewarded with positive feedback on their contribution, either during or after the discussion. The teacher could say, "Debbie made a good point just now. Has anyone else had that experience?" If the teacher doesn't want to intervene during the discussion, a comment of appreciation for the student's contribution right after class can still be helpful.

The teacher should try to discourage students who are talking too much and not letting others take part. Avoiding eye contact may work to some extent. Sometimes one must simply be blunt and say, "We've been hearing a lot from Carol, now let's hear what the rest of you think."

Part of the leader's role is to direct the discussion between and among members of the group; comments should not be addressed directly to the leader. If every student looks at and talks to the leader, he or she is going to be much too verbal, having to respond to or redirect each comment. Instead, the leader should make it clear that if Student A has something to say about what Student B has just contributed, Student A should address the comment to Student B. The leader's interventions should only be to support the group process and occasionally introduce comments or questions that will move the discussion along and accomplish the objectives.

In the course of the discussion, the teacher may need to clarify students' statements in order to avoid misinterpretation and confusion. Such clarification should be used sparingly but is sometimes necessary to facilitate the discussion. Rewording what a student has said may also help students learn the art of clear self-expression. If rewording a student's comment seems demeaning, the teacher might instead ask the student to give an example of what he or she is talking about.

It is perfectly acceptable and sometimes desirable to have periods of silence in a discussion. Although students, and some teachers, are uncomfortable with silence, it gives everyone in the group a chance to think about what has been said and to organize his or her thoughts. During a lull in the talking, a shy student may get up the nerve to say something.

The group leader also has the responsibility to summarize when appropriate. A summary may be in order when moving from one aspect of a topic to a new aspect, or it may be saved for the end of the discussion. Summaries can help put the discussion into perspective and show how objectives have been met. An example of a typical summary statement is "You have all shared your opinions and experiences and insights into the problem of substance abuse among nurses. We have seen the scope of the problem and felt its seriousness. But I think we've also gained some ideas on what can be done to help impaired nurses . . ."

These are but some of the techniques instructors can use to lead effective discussions. Experienced teachers also develop their own techniques that work for them. Although not every discussion will meet your expectations, with conscientious planning and leading, most class discussions can be fruitful.

Advantages of the Discussion Method

Many of the advantages of discussion are linked to its purposes. Thus the advantages include practice in problem solving, training in self-expression and critical thinking, and increased familiarity with the group process. In addition, the student is placed in an active role, and positive correlations have been found between active participation in learning and the retention and recall of information (see Chapter 2).

Gaut and Blainey believe that the main advantage of the discussion method is the message that it conveys: "Wanted: an exchange of ideas, opinions, reactions, and conclusions from all participants in this learning environment" (1982; 75). Students feel that their knowledge is valued and that they have something worthwhile to teach each other. When the discussion is handled well by the leader, participants receive positive reinforcement for their contributions and their self-esteem is bolstered.

Disadvantages of the Discussion Method

One drawback to class discussions is that they are time consuming. There is no doubt that discussion is an inefficient way to communicate information. Methods such as lecture or computer-assisted instruction are superior in terms of time efficiency. Also, formal discussions usually require more than an hour of class time, so if class sessions are only one hour long, effective discussions may not take place.

Discussion may also be less effective if the class is large, because not all members can become active participants. Experts usually advocate discussion groups of 5 to 20 students (Gall & Gall, 1976). With classes of more than 20 students, the faculty member may have to assign students to smaller discussion groups. The disadvantage to this procedure is that the teacher cannot be the discussion leader or moderator for all students.

We have all participated in discussion groups where one person or a few people monopolized the discussion. This is always a danger of the discussion method unless the group leader controls the situation. If only a few members are participating, the others are relegated to a passive learning role, and learning is especially inhibited if the vocal few are not contributing valuable viewpoints or conclusions.

Finally, discussion is usually valuable only if students have come to class prepared. The contribution of uninformed opinions and misinformation benefits no one, and the discussion becomes simply a sharing of each other's ignorance.

Research on Discussion

Most research on the discussion method has compared it with other methods, particularly lectures. One body of research has, however, dealt solely with discussion: research concerned with discussion and attitude change. Gall and Gall (1976) summarized studies conducted between 1947 and 1973 that consistently found attitude changes resulting from discussion. Discussion was responsible for inducing mothers to give their children orange juice and cod liver oil, students to volunteer for experiments, and parents to change their attitudes toward mental retardation.

Several writers have summarized some of the early research on the effectiveness of lecture versus discussion. Gayles (1966) reported the following findings from studies conducted between 1942 and 1959:

1. The lecture method was better for immediate recall and for superior students, but discussion was better for delayed recall and for weaker students.

2. Achievement of course content was about the same with either method.

3. Lecture was superior to discussion on a test of facts, but discussion was superior for teaching problem solving.

4. More positive attitude changes occurred with discussion than with lecture.

McKeachie (1969), summarizing the results of 15 researchers who worked in the 1940s and '50s, reported that slightly more than half of the studies found lecture to be more effective than discussion when a factual examination was used as the outcome criterion. However, discussion was superior with higher-level cognitive outcomes and with outcomes of changed attitudes and increased motivation.

In 1953, Bloom studied the effectiveness of lecture and discussion by using a technique termed *stimulated recall*. Lecture classes and discussion classes were taped, and within 48 hours the tapes were replayed to the students, who were asked to report the thoughts they had been having at various points throughout the original class. It was found that during lectures students had significantly more thoughts irrelevant to the point of the class than did students in discussion groups. Also, in the lecture classes students had thoughts indicating a minimal level of attentiveness, just keeping the main ideas in mind, whereas in the discussion classes significantly more thoughts involved attempts to find solutions to problems and synthesis of ideas about the subject. In general, the lecture classes were relatively successful in holding students' attention, but discussion classes were more successful in evoking higher-level thinking.

More recently, Canter and Gallatin (1974) studied student preferences for either method. They believed that past studies showing that students preferred lectures over discussions might have been influenced by the fact that course examinations are usually better prepared for by studying lecture notes than by trying to recall discussions. Students therefore feel more confident of doing well on an examination if the material has been taught by means of lectures. When the researchers studied preferences in a case where no examination was given on the class material, they found no significant differences in preference for either method.

In 1977 Watts reported a comparison study of lecture, discussion, and audiovisual methods. A unit on human sexuality was taught by each method. Knowledge gain was greatest in the lecture class. No method was found to be superior for changing attitudes.

As with any research topic, conflicting results occur and variables are not always well controlled. But a great deal of evidence has accumulated to support the practice of using the discussion method for teaching problem solving and higher levels of cognitive learning and for changing attitudes. It is also a popular method with students and can be used to increase motivation. More research needs to be done on ways and means of making the discussion method as effective as possible in meeting these objectives.

Questioning

Asking questions is such an integral part of teaching that many teachers take it for granted. They ask questions to assess student comprehension but don't give much thought to using questioning as a teaching strategy. Questions are essential to teaching effective thinking processes—teaching students how to use knowledge. If students are to be active learners, they must seek the answers to questions, learn how to process information, and discover how to ask the right questions for themselves.

Educators must learn to use questions that will achieve their objectives. This is not an easy task. It is easy to ask questions that call for factual responses and test only recall. It is much more difficult to design questions that will stimulate higher-level thinking.

Awareness of the efficacy of questioning as a teaching method seems to have begun with Socrates. In the Socratic method, the teacher asks a series of questions that are designed to first make the student aware of his or her ignorance and then to reason out the truth about an issue. It is an application of the discovery method of learning and as such is time consuming, especially since it is best conducted with only one student at a time. Although few today follow the Socratic pattern, instructors would do well to put more emphasis on questioning as a means of teaching reasoning and thinking processes.

Functions of Questioning

The use of questioning places students in the role of active learners. They are asked to recall, to form links between previously isolated information, to analyze statements or beliefs, to evaluate the worth of ideas, to speculate about what would happen "if." As questions are asked, students start to mentally formulate answers if they think they may be called on in class. They cannot just sit and daydream unless they are willing to appear stupid in the eyes of their classmates. Students may become excited as they realize that they can come up with the answers to questions and that they are discovering valuable information.

Motivation to learn can increase as students hear questions for which they would like to know the answers. The teacher may pose a problem or dilemma and raise questions, and students are motivated to come up with solutions. Knowledgeable teachers use questions to guide students' thought processes in a certain direction. Suppose a teacher wants to explore the chain of infection in hospitals. Her first question might be "Why is there a higher rate of infection among hospitalized patents than patients who are ill at home?" This might be followed by "Yes, patients can get infections from each other, but what about some other sources of infection?" Then, "Contaminated equipment can be responsible, too. Is there anything else?" After exploring all of the sources of infection, the instructor would try to elicit the concept of a *reservoir* of pathogens by asking, "What term could you use to describe the existence of a ready supply of pathogens in the hospital?" Questions could continue that would elicit the other links in the chain of infection. In so guiding the students' thinking on a subject, the teacher extends their knowledge, encouraging them to think logically and deepening their understanding of a subject.

Questions can be used to assess a baseline of knowledge—to find out what the class already knows about a subject. They can also help the teacher to assess understanding and retention of information. If the students are having trouble grasping concepts or following the teacher's thought process, questioning can quickly uncover their problems.

Questioning can also be used to review content. If the instructor wants to spend 5 minutes at the beginning of class reviewing content from the previous class, it might be more enlightening to do so by means of questions rather than lecturing.

Questioning can also serve as positive reinforcement for students. Indicating that a student's answer was correct or insightful provides feedback not only that he or she understood the material and was using good thought processes but also that the answer was appreciated. A wrong answer deserves careful handling so that the feedback is correct but not devastating. A teacher might respond to a wrong answer by saying, "There is some truth in what you are saying, Linda, but let me clarify one point" or "Your reasoning is good, Steve, but your conclusion is faulty."

Levels of Questions

Questions can be formulated that stimulate specific levels of cognitive activity in students. Educators have devised many classification systems for questions. Here we will examine a few of the most common classifications.

One system divides questions into three types: concrete, abstract, and creative (Carner, 1963). *Concrete* questions elicit answers based on concrete thinking. These questions are low level and call for facts, literal meanings, and simple ideas. "Who," "what," "where," and "when" questions fit in this category. *Abstract* questions require students to go beyond isolated facts to generalize, classify, and draw conclusions about pieces of data. Questions starting with "how" and "why" call for abstract thinking. *Creative* questions demand the reorganization of concepts into new patterns and may require both abstract and concrete thinking. Questions such as "What would happen if . . . ?" and "How else could you . . . ?" require creative thinking.

Another classification system has four levels: cognitive-memory questions, convergent questions, divergent questions, and evaluative questions (Hyman, 1974). *Cognitive-memory* questions require only low-level thinking; recall and recognition of facts fit in this category. *Convergent* questions demand that students analyze and integrate data; reasoning is required as well as recall. An example of a convergent question is "Explain why neuromuscular hyperactivity occurs in hypoparathyroidism." *Divergent* questions require students to generate new ideas, draw implications, or formulate a new perspective on a topic. Divergent thinking would be used to answer the question "What would happen if we tried . . . ?" *Evaluative* questions deal with judgment, assessment, and valuing. This level of cognitive activity is evident in such questions as "What do you think of . . . ?" and "How would you rate . . . ?"

The most popular classification system is based on Bloom's taxonomy (Bloom, 1956). Although the taxonomy was written to classify educational objectives, it nicely explains levels of questions. Thus, many educators refer to questions that elicit thinking at the levels of knowledge, comprehension, application, analysis, synthesis, and evaluation. Table 4-1 lists the cognitive activity and

Table 4-1   Question Classification

Category	Cognitive Activity Required	Key Concepts	Sample Question Words
1. KNOWLEDGE	RECALL Questions, regardless of complexity, can be answered by simple recall of previously learned material	Memory Repetition Description Knowledge	What; When; Who; Which; Define; Describe; Identify; List; Name; Recall; Show; State; How; Indicate; Tell; Yes/No questions; e.g. Did? Was? Is?
2. COMPREHENSION	UNDERSTANDING Questions can be answered by merely restating and reorganizing material in a rather literal manner to show that the student understands the essential meaning.	Explanation Comparison Illustration	Compare; Contrast; Conclude; Demonstrate; Differentiate; Predict; Reorder; Which; Why; Distinguish; Estimate; Explain; Extend; Extrapolate; Rearrange; Rephrase; Inform; What; Fill in; Give an example of; Illustrate; Relate; Tell in your own words
3. APPLICATION	SOLVING Questions involve problem solving in *new* situations with minimal identification or prompting of the appropriate rules, principles, or concepts	Solution Application	Apply; Build; Construct; Solve; Test; Consider; Demonstrate (in a new situation); How would; Check out
4. ANALYSIS	EXPLORATION OF REASONING Questions require the student to break an idea into its component parts for logical analysis, facts, opinions, logical conclusions, etc.	Induction Deduction Logical	Support your; What assumptions; What reasons; Does the evidence support the conclusion; What does the patient seem to believe about; What words indicate bias or emotion; What behaviors

Table 4-1, continued   Question Classification

Category	Cognitive Activity Required	Key Concepts	Sample Question Words
5. SYNTHESIS	CREATING Questions require students to combine ideas into a statement, plan, product, etc. that is new for them.	Productive Thinking Novelty	Write; Think of a way; Create; Propose a plan; Put together; Suggest; Develop; Make up; Formulate a solution; Synthesize; Derive
6. EVALUATION	JUDGING Questions require students to make a judgment about something using some criteria or standard by making their judgment principles, or concepts	Judgment Selection	Choose; Evaluate in terms of; Decide; Judge; Select on the basis of; Which would you consider; Defend; What is the most appropriate; For what reasons do you favor; Which policy

Source: Craig JL, Page G: The questioning skills of nursing instructors. *J Nurs Educ* 1981; 20:20.

key concepts at each level, as well as some sample question words. Here are some examples of questions at each cognitive level:

Knowledge

> What is the definition of glaucoma?
>
> At what age do infants begin to crawl?

Comprehension

> What does the nursing process have in common with the scientific method?
>
> Why does intravenous tubing have to be free of air?

Application

> Given these arterial blood gas results, what nursing interventions are needed?
>
> How would you get a blood pressure reading on a person with third-degree burns of all extremities?

Analysis

> What is the major premise behind Kübler-Ross's theory of death and dying?
>
> What data would you need to support this nursing diagnosis?

Synthesis

> Given all of the data in this case study, what nursing diagnoses can be developed?
>
> Think of a way that we could research the relationship between those variables.

Evaluation

> Of the two possible nursing interventions in this situation, which would be more appropriate?

Which leadership style would make the best use of the employees' abilities?

You can see that Bloom's taxonomy really includes the commonalities of all the classification systems. Because most educators are familiar with Bloom's work, it is a useful way to categorize levels of questions.

Keep in mind that a single question could be placed in several categories, depending on the context. The example given for the comprehension level of "Why does intravenous tubing have to be free of air?" could be a knowledge question if the student had previously been told why and is now simply recalling it. It becomes a comprehension question if the student has been taught only in general terms about the effects of air in the circulatory system. It could also fit at the analysis level if the subject had not previously been discussed at all but the student has a physics and physiology background and is expected to analyze the question in terms of known principles of physics and hemodynamics. Teachers cannot always know at what level a student is answering a question because they lack knowledge of the student's background in the subject.

Types of Questions

Besides varying the cognitive levels of questions, instructors can choose from seven types of questions to achieve different purposes.

1. *Yes/no questions.* With yes/no questions, the teacher asks a question such as "Do emotional crises always have negative outcomes?" and the student is simply asked to affirm or deny the idea in the question or to say "I don't know." Yes/no questions can be used to open a further line of questioning or to simply assess whether the teacher has the students' attention.

2. *Cue questions.* When the teacher wants a student to further explain an answer, he or she may use a lead or cue such as "Can you explain that?" or "Can you tell us a little more about why you have taken that position?" Such questions are helpful in assessing students' comprehension and thought processes.

3. *Multiple-choice questions.* Such questions can be oral as well as written. "Is NPH insulin a short-, intermediate-, or long-acting insulin?" is an oral multiple-choice question. If you use this

type, be careful not to include too many options, or it becomes confusing. Multiple-choice questions test recall and can be used to begin a discussion.

4. *Open-ended questions.* This broad category encompasses all questions that require students to construct an answer, just like short-answer test questions. Questions such as "When should fetal monitoring be used?" and "Can you explain how a volume-cycled respirator works?" are open-ended questions.

5. *Discussion-stimulating questions.* Once discussion about a subject has been initiated, the teacher can use various questions to promote it. Questions such as "What do the rest of you think of that statement?" "Do you agree with John's position?" and "Has anyone else had that experience?" help to move the discussion along.

6. *Questions that guide problem solving.* A teacher needs to phrase and sequence questions carefully in order to guide students through problem-solving thinking. Typical questions might be "What information do we need before we can solve this problem? "What other options do we have?" and "What would be the effect of that action?"

7. *Rhetorical questions.* It is sometimes appropriate to ask questions for which you expect no answers at the time. Such questions can be used to stimulate thinking in the class and may guide students into asking some of their own questions as they study a topic. What is used as a rhetorical question in one session may become a source of discussion in a later session.

There is value in asking students a variety of types of questions at different cognitive levels. They need to be able to think and respond in all ways. Unfortunately, as research points out, most teachers ask questions primarily at the lower cognitive levels. In view of the high-level thinking required of nurses in most work situations, it would seem more beneficial to accustom students to formulating a higher percentage of answers at the application through evaluation levels. It may be that certain types of questions would be more effective than others in teaching nursing; further research in this area might be enlightening.

Gall (1970) also suggests that research into the topic of follow-up questions is needed. A teacher may ask a knowledge-level question such as "What is bowel retraining?" Follow-ups to this question might be "What methods can be used to retrain bowel habits?" "What are the physiological principles underlying these procedures?" and "For which patients might bowel retraining be most successful?" Because follow-up questions can lift the student to higher cognitive levels, it would be helpful to know whether the sequence of the follow-up questions makes any difference in helping the student to develop his or her thinking abilities. Both the level of and sequencing of follow-up questions may have an impact on learning.

Questioning Techniques

Incorporating good questioning procedures into classes requires planning and forethought. The first prerequisite is to establish an atmosphere in which students feel fairly relaxed and free to ask and answer questions. It takes some time, maybe a few class sessions, before the students decide that the teacher really wants them to talk and will not humiliate them if they come up with wrong answers.

Another aspect of planning is preparing some questions ahead of time. If your questions are to meet the objectives for the class session and be at the appropriate cognitive level, they require careful preparation. Not every question can be planned, because it is difficult to tell how students will respond and which channels their answers will take, but the introductory questions for major topics should be planned.

Both the prepared questions and those formulated in the midst of discussion must be stated clearly and specifically. A vague or poorly worded question will probably elicit silent stares. Research has revealed that the clarity of teachers' questions does have an effect on the clarity of students' answers and the level of learning outcomes (Wenk & Menges, 1985). A question like "What are the legal principles that should guide your nursing care?" is so broad and nonspecific that students would probably be unsure of how to answer. Instead, the same objectives might be achieved with the question "You read about the legal principle of *respondeat superior*. Can you give me an example of a malpractice suit in which this principle applies?"

The teacher's response to a student's answer is very important. A nod, a smile, or a comment that shows the answer is correct and appreciated are all appropriate. The instructor should be careful, though, not to give too rapid a reward. If the teacher immediately says, "Right" after the first student gives an answer, students who are slower thinkers may be prevented from formulating and offering their own answers (Napell, 1976). Instead, the teacher should allow a few seconds of silence while looking around at the other students or should ask, "Can anyone else add to that answer?"

Another valuable practice is to tolerate a few seconds of silence when there is no immediate response to a question. The instructor should avoid jumping right in to answer the question, especially if it requires complex thinking. Research data indicate that teachers generally allow only 1 second before repeating the question or calling on another student (Hyman, 1974). When teachers increase their waiting time to 3 to 5 seconds, the number and length of appropriate responses increase, and a greater variety of students enter the discussion. There should be a limit to one's patience, however. If after 5 seconds the students do not answer, the teacher should either rephrase the question or acknowledge it to be too difficult and move on. The instructor should avoid asking too many questions that are too difficult for the students. No useful purpose is served in asking students a lot of questions that they can't possibly answer.

A problem among some teachers is always trying to top a student's answer. It is tempting to add a little more information to every answer to show the students what a truly correct response should have included or what an expert would have said. Some teachers may even wait for several responses and then say "You are all close, but . . ." No doubt there are times when one must flesh out students' answers, but teachers should avoid setting themselves up as the ultimate word on every subject and on every occasion. This kind of behavior is insidious; a teacher may never know that he or she is doing it unless someone points it out, but it has definite negative effects on student behavior. This habit dampens discussion and discourages student openness and risk taking.

Making judgmental responses to students' answers is another teacher behavior that should be avoided (Eaton et al, 1977). An instructor who asks for student opinions must be prepared to respect them. Even if students offer unsolicited opinions, they should not be put down because the teacher doesn't agree or doesn't value their viewpoint. There is a place for teachers to share their opinions and values; in fact, they must pass on professional and moral values to future nurses. But students' opinions must also be respected, especially as they relate to their personal lives. If a student voices an attitude contrary to what is expected in professional nursing, the student should not be snubbed; rather, the educator must enlist teaching strategies such as discussions, role playing, and so on to help shape desirable attitudes.

Stimulating Student Questioning

One of the outcomes of questioning as a teaching method should be that students learn how to ask questions. In fact, students should be rewarded just as much or more for asking good questions as they are for giving good answers.

Teachers can stimulate student questioning by guiding their thinking along a path that will lead to the development of questions and hypotheses about a subject. But this guidance must take place in an atmosphere where it is safe to take risks and to ask questions that might seem stupid. Indeed, teachers should actually invite questions.

Instructors also have to monitor their teaching behaviors to ensure that they are not unknowingly discouraging questions. Nonverbally, teachers may indicate their unwillingness to entertain questions or their dislike of the questions asked by avoiding eye contact, blatantly ignoring raised hands, or appearing distracted or impatient while a student is talking. A teacher may also use seemingly innocuous statements such as "Can you hold that question until I'm finished?" "You're getting ahead of the topic; we'll deal with that later" or "Unless anyone has any burning questions or brilliant insights, we'll end here." Although any of these statements may be necessary at times, their habitual use will soon convey the message that the teacher doesn't really want to be interrupted with questions, and any questions that *are* asked had better be good. Nothing is more apt to discourage the average student from venturing a question. Being aware of such behavior can help teachers change their verbal and nonverbal patterns.

Research on Questioning

Although a considerable amount of research has been done on the use of questions in education, much of it has suffered from methodologic problems and most has been done at the grammar school or high school levels. As you will see in the studies that follow, results are often conflicting.

Three studies in which the cognitive levels of teachers' questions were investigated did show similar results. In 1967 Davis and Tinsley studied 44 secondary-school student teachers and found that more "memory" questions were asked than all other questions combined. Over half of the student teachers asked no questions at the application, analysis, or synthesis levels.

Two nurse educators analyzed the levels of questions asked in clinical conferences of a baccalaureate nursing program (Scholdra & Quiring, 1973). They found that both faculty and students asked 98.94% lower-level questions (especially recall and comprehension) in spite of the fact that the objectives of the conferences were to stimulate higher-level thinking.

When Barnes (1983) observed 40 college professors randomly selected from four undergraduate institutions, she discovered that the majority of questions were at the lowest cognitive level, and a small portion of most classes was devoted to questioning. Another interesting finding was that 31.93% of all questions elicited no student response.

Three more researchers looked at the relationship between cognitive levels of questions and student outcomes. In 1967 Hunkins (cited in Gall, 1970) designed an experiment in which one group of sixth-grade students were taught social studies with questions at the knowledge level, while a second group of students were taught by means of questions at the analysis and evaluation levels. On a specially formulated posttest, the analysis/evaluation group performed significantly better on the entire test but especially on the sections that contained application and evaluation questions.

Ryan (1973) selected a sample of 104 fifth and sixth graders who were studying geography. He formed a "low-questioning group" in which the teacher used questions at the recall level and a "high-questioning group" taught by questions above the recall level. The students later took two multiple-choice tests, one to measure low-level (recall) achievement, the other to measure higher-than-recall achievement. The high-questioning group performed better on both tests.

A third study of sixth graders was conducted by Martin (1979), who found that increasing the frequency of higher-order questions resulted in increases in the frequency of higher-order student responses but had no effect on student achievement on specially designed test questions.

Other authors have summarized groups of studies investigating the effectiveness of questioning as a teaching method. Winne (1979) reviewed 18 experimental studies dealing with the effectiveness of teachers using relatively more higher-level cognitive questions versus relatively fewer higher-level questions. He found no solid evidence that the predominant use of higher-level questions enhanced student achievement. Redfield and Rousseau (1981) used the meta-analytic technique to synthesize the findings of 20 experimental studies of the influence of question levels on student achievement. They included the 18 studies reviewed by Winne. These researchers found an overall positive effect on student achievement with the predominant use of higher-level cognitive questions. The difference in research techniques used by Winne versus Redfield and Rousseau apparently accounts for the differing results.

Over the years various groups of educators have attempted to develop inservice programs for improving teachers' questioning abilities. Results have fairly consistently demonstrated that questioning practices can be improved and that the cognitive level of questions can be raised with specific training (Gall, 1970; Craig & Page, 1981).

A great deal of research still needs to be done in this area. We need more studies with tighter methodology before we can say with confidence that higher-level questions result in greater student achievement, and we need to find out what kinds of learning outcomes can best be achieved through questioning.

The Interactive Lecture

It should be clear by this point that the techniques of lecture, discussion, and questioning can be effectively blended together into an interactive lecture, utilizing the advantages of all the methods and reducing their disadvantages.

Class time can be logically and efficiently divided into sections for lecture, informal discussion, questioning, more lecturing, and so on. In this way subject matter is presented for discussion, problem solving can take place, and questions can stimulate student thinking and clarify difficult points. Students become periodically active in the class, which eliminates some of the objections to pure lecturing.

Changing tactics every 15 to 20 minutes may also help to recapture students' attention at points when it naturally seems to wander. The class becomes more interesting and, it is to be hoped, more memorable. Although pure lecture, discussion, and questioning sessions can and should be used at times, the interactive lecture is a good alternative that can achieve many learning objectives.

I have saved the discussion of one more research study for this

point because it illustrates what goes on in many college classrooms in which the interactive lecture format is used. It gives
insight into the ways students may operate in such a setting and
has implications for the manner in which teachers should conduct
such a class.

Karp and Yoels (1976) collected data from ten classes in a
northeastern university by means of observation and questionnaires. Their findings include:

1. About 95% of the students said they could tell very early in the
   semester whether a professor really wanted discussion in class.

2. Questions and comments by the teacher accounted for 88% of
   the classroom interactions.

3. In classes with fewer than 40 students, 4 or 5 students accounted for most student interactions; in classes of more than
   40 students, 2 or 3 students accounted for the majority of interactions.

4. Some 10% of classroom interactions involved cases in which
   students responded to questions or comments of other students.

5. Of all classroom interactions, only about 10% were questions
   directed by the teacher to a particular student.

6. The reasons students ranked most important for not getting
   involved in discussion were "not doing the assigned reading,"
   "ignorance of subject matter," and "my ideas are not well
   enough formulated."

7. About 42% of students said that the possibility that they would
   appear unintelligent in the eyes of other students was an important factor in keeping them from talking in class; 80% of the
   teachers thought that this was probably an important factor in
   preventing discussion.

8. Five minutes or less of each 50-minute class period was accounted for by student talking.

These findings, if typical (and they seem to be in my experience), indicate that teachers need to use more of the techniques
mentioned in this chapter for encouraging student participation,
getting students more actively involved in class, and holding stu-

dents accountable for class preparation, perhaps by asking more questions of specific individuals. Successful interactive lectures require a significant amount of meaningful interaction between students and teachers.

References

Barnes CP: Questioning in college classrooms. Pages 61–81 in: *Studies of College Teaching*. Ellner CL, Barnes CP (editors): Heath, 1983.

Bloom BS: Thought processes in lectures and discussions. *J General Educ* 1953; 7:160–169.

Bloom BS (editor): *Taxonomy of Educational Objectives Handbook I: Cognitive Domain*. Longman, 1956.

Canter F, Gallatin J: Lecture versus discussion as related to students' personality factors. *Improving College and University Teaching* 1974; 22:111–112, 116.

Carner RL: Levels of questioning. *Education* 1963; 83:546–550.

Craig JL, Page G: The questioning skills of nursing instructors. *J Nurs Educ* (May) 1981; 20:18–23.

Davis OL, Tinsley DC: Cognitive objectives revealed by classroom questions asked by social studies teachers. *Peabody J Educ* (July) 1967; 45:21–26.

Davis RJ: Secrets of master lecturers. *Improving College and University Teaching* 1965; 13:150–151.

Eaton S, Davis GL, Benner PE: Discussion stoppers in teaching. *Nurs Outlook* 1977; 25:578–583.

Gall MD: The use of questions in teaching. *Rev Educ Res* 1970; 40:707–721.

Gall MD, Gall JP: The discussion method. Pages 166–216 in: *The Psychology of Teaching Methods*. Gage NL (editor). University of Chicago Press, 1976.

Gaut DA, Blainey CG: The lecture approach to teaching nursing—method or habit? *Nurs Health Care* 1982; 3:73–82.

Gayles AR: Lecture vs. discussion. *Improving College and University Teaching* 1966; 14:95–99.

Gotesky R: The lecture and critical thinking. *Educ Forum* 1966; 30:179–187.

Heller MP: Learning through lectures. *Clearing House* 1962; 37:99–100.

Hyman RT: *Ways of Teaching* 2d ed. Lippincott, 1974.

Karp DA, Yoels WC: The college classroom: some observations on the meanings of student participation. *Sociology and Social Research* 1976; 60:421–439.

MacManaway LA: Using lecture scripts. *Universities Quarterly* 1968; 22:327–336.

Marr JN et al: The contribution of the lecture to college teaching. *J Educ Psych* 1960; 51:277–284.

Martin J: Effects of teacher higher-order questions on student process and product variables in a single-classroom study. *J Educ Res* 1979; 72:183–187.

McKeachie WJ: *Teaching Tips: a Guidebook for the Beginning College Teacher.* Heath, 1969.

McLeish J: The lecture method. Pages 252–301 in: *The Psychology of Teaching Methods.* Gage NL (editor). University of Chicago Press, 1976.

Napell SM: Six common nonfacilitating teaching behaviors. *Contemporary Educ* 1976; 47:79–82.

Palmer SE: The art of lecturing: a few simple ideas can help teachers improve their skills. *Chronicle of Higher Educ* (April) 1983; 26:19–20.

Redfield DL, Rousseau EW: A meta-analysis of experimental research on teacher questioning behavior. *Rev Educ Res* 1981; 51:237–245.

Ryan FL: Differentiated effects of levels of questioning on student achievement. *J Exper Educ* (Spring) 1973; 41:63–67.

Schoen JR: Use of consciousness sampling to study teaching methods. *J Educ Res* 1970; 63:387–390.

Scholdra JD, Quiring JD: The level of questions posed by nursing educators. *J Nurs Educ* (Aug) 1973; 12:15–19.

Stuart J, Rutherford RJD: Medical student concentration during lectures. *Lancet* 1978; 2:514–516.

Thomas EJ: The variation of memory with time for information appearing during a lecture. *Studies in Adult Educ* 1972; 4:57–62.

Watts PR: Comparison of three human sexuality teaching methods used in university health classes. *Res Quarterly* (March) 1977; 48:187–190.

Winne PH: Experiments relating teachers' use of higher cognitive questions to student achievement. *Rev Educ Res* 1979; 49:13–50.

Wenk VA, Menges RJ: Using classroom questions appropriately. *Nurse Educator* (March/April) 1985; 10:19–24.

Chapter 5

Seminar, Brainstorming, Debate

The strategies of seminar, brainstorming, and debate have much in common with the discussion method, yet each is also a distinct entity. This chapter elaborates on the use of all three and explains how they mesh with discussion techniques.

Seminar

Seminars have historically been defined as small groups of students engaged in research who meet with a professor to discuss common problems and pursuits. Today the term *seminar* is used more broadly to encompass small groups that meet to discuss the results of library or empirical research. This broad definition serves as a rubric for the varied types of seminars that may be conducted.

Generally seminars are composed of 10 to 20 students who individually or in small subgroups investigate pertinent topics, analyze them, and draw some conclusions. The topics are presented orally to the larger seminar group, which further analyzes, critiques, and applies the topic.

Purpose of the Seminar Method

The purpose of a seminar goes beyond discussion of important topics—that purpose could be achieved by a general discussion group. Rather, the seminar strategy is designed to teach and develop group process and leadership skills. It is for this reason that seminars are mostly, if not totally, led by students.

Nurses are, in the course of their work, often involved in organizing and leading groups. They may be a part of an agency committee; they often do group teaching or counseling; they may lead support groups or other community groups. Nursing students must have practice in the role of professional group leader and in analyzing and critiquing other people in that role. The seminar is a logical vehicle for learning about this role.

While students in a seminar are learning group process and leadership, they are also learning how to think, investigate, and convey ideas clearly, as is true of the discussion method in general. They are also learning some content, but that is secondary to learning the process skills. The seminar is not an efficient way to teach content.

Uses of the Seminar Method

Originally, seminars were used only at the graduate school level. Now they are used in undergraduate curricula, especially at the junior and senior year levels, at which point students have mastered a great deal of nursing content and are more prepared for a leadership role. Seminars can also be used as a teaching method in inservice education.

The small enrollments in seminar courses are justified by the purposes of the seminar. It would not make sense to use lecture or computer-assisted instruction for such groups; the small-group time is best used for close, intense work with a professor and with peers.

The topics covered in seminar courses vary greatly. Many nursing programs have a senior seminar, but a close look will reveal wide disparity in content. Some schools focus on current issues in nursing, such as entry level, unionism, and euthanasia. Others include topics about the professional role, such as working with other professionals, accountability, and legal issues. Still others include clinical content, such as community health and related issues (Anderson, 1980). Cooper (1979) has suggested that seminars are useful as a method for providing continuing education programs such as reports of research in progress.

The content of the course should be something that can be mastered fairly quickly by students, since they will be leading the seminars and will be the supposed "experts." It would be inappropriate to bring in a lot of clinical content that could only be mastered after months or years of clinical practice. On the other hand, a topic like euthanasia, although very broad, can be narrowed down and researched quite effectively with a few weeks of preparation.

Seminar Techniques

I have taught undergraduate senior seminars that focused on exploring current issues in nursing and developing group leadership skills. My techniques are by no means unique, so I will describe them here as a basic model. Creative teachers could use the basic techniques and expand them to meet the needs of their setting.

In my 2-hour seminars, teams of two students were assigned to lead each session. They could choose a topic from a suggested list or could develop another topic if it met the course objectives. The first student-led seminar did not take place for at least 3 weeks. I used those first few weeks to work with the pairs of students in developing their topics and their leadership role. Vande Zande (1987), when conducting a similar seminar class, used the first few weeks for teacher-led seminars on group process and group leadership.

Students in my groups had to develop a bibliography and indicate one or two required readings for the rest of the class. It is essential that advance readings be required or the seminar group will not be prepared to fully discuss the issue, and the seminar will disintegrate into a lecture by the student leaders or, worse, simply a sharing of uninformed opinions. The bibliography was distributed to all members of the seminar group at least 1 week in advance.

A variety of techniques were available to seminar leaders. They could introduce their topic with a lecture or audiovisuals (if they were brief). Some used overhead transparencies and tapes of interviews with experts on the topic. At some point in the seminar, the leaders were required to talk about the role of the nurse or the nursing profession in relation to the issue. Some leaders presented this aspect themselves; others asked the rest of the group to synthesize what they had already discussed in the seminar and to formulate some answers.

The seminar leaders were held accountable for involving the whole group in discussion. They brought some prepared questions to stimulate discussion, and they were supposed to direct the discussion and keep it on track. Obviously, students varied in their abilities as group leaders. Some dominated the entire discussion, while others abdicated their role to a stronger group member. Most were able to apply leadership and group dynamics principles well, however.

The role of the teacher in this configuration varies. I chose to participate very little in the actual seminars. I found during the first few that I got too caught up in being a member of the discussion group, barely biding my time until I could say something. By doing so, I was not paying enough attention to evaluating what the leaders and other students were doing and saying. Subsequently, I confined my role to coaching before and after the seminars and using seminar time primarily to evaluate the process going on in the room. Vande Zande (1987) relates that her role as teacher in the seminars was to be a discussion member. Each faculty member can develop the role somewhat differently. A staff development teacher might choose an active role in the discussion since she or he is often seen as a colleague in the group rather than as an authority figure and since evaluation of the participants may not be necessary.

I evaluated both seminar leaders and participants each week. Evaluation of group participation is desirable if you want all students to come prepared and to take part in the discussion. In addition, I had each student, leader or participant, fill out a self-evaluation each week. Another option is to have the group members evaluate the leaders. All this evaluation is somewhat cumbersome, but I found it necessary in order to arrive at fair grades, since almost all the work in the course was presented orally.

Graduate research seminars would require different teaching techniques because the purposes are different. The objectives of graduate-level seminars are usually to help individual students develop a research proposal and develop critical thinking abilities with regard to research. One student presents his or her ideas for a research proposal and the others critique the ideas and attempt to solve some of the difficulties foreseen. The teacher takes an active role in helping to guide students' thinking. Little formal evaluation takes place in a seminar of this type. Students often receive a "pass" grade simply for attending and developing their proposal as far as possible.

Seminars are valuable if they are used correctly. The relative expense of running a class for only 10 or 15 students is only justified, however, if the seminar format is adhered to and if students achieve the desired learning outcomes.

Brainstorming

Brainstorming was originally developed by Alex Osborn (1957) for use in the business world. He wanted to stimulate the creativity of members of an advertising agency to generate new ideas in an uninhibited atmosphere. He encouraged groups of people to think of all possible ways of looking at an idea or all possible solutions to a problem. Osborn believed that group members could think more creatively when exposed to the ideas of others and that premature application of limitations and criticism to ideas only serves to limit creativity. As a result of these beliefs, he formulated four rules or guidelines for brainstorming:

1. Criticism and judgment are to be withheld until all ideas have been generated.

2. All ideas should be expressed even if they seem wild.

3. Quantity of ideas rather than quality is sought.

4. Combinations and transformations of ideas are desirable.

Uses of Brainstorming

Brainstorming can be used in the classroom or in clinical conferences. Whenever a potential or actual patient problem arises, learners can be asked to brainstorm solutions. They can also use this method to arrive at possible solutions to professional problems such as the inaccurate image of nursing, burnout among nurses, and soaring malpractice insurance rates. Not only does brainstorming become a part of problem solving, it becomes a route to creative thinking. Students need to be taught how to think creatively, to expand their options, and to break out of narrow channels of thought.

Brainstorming Techniques

Brainstorming can be used in any discussion group. Smaller groups tend to work best, as all ideas can be expressed. The teacher introduces the topic and the procedures to be followed. He or she states the ground rules and the time limit, if there is one. The teacher is usually the best person to be the recorder of ideas (on paper, chalkboard, or tape). If about 20 minutes is going to be devoted to the exercise, about one-third of that time should be given to individuals to come up with their ideas; the remaining time can be used for the group to exchange ideas, build on the ideas expressed, and finally, to evaluate the potential effectiveness of the ideas. Although evaluation is not actually a part of brainstorming, it is a necessary follow-up. Getting the ideas out in the open is wonderful, but some of the ideas will indeed be wild and of no practical value; others that seem ridiculous at first may have hidden merit.

A brief example will serve to show how brainstorming can be used. Suppose that a learner has a patient with Alzheimer's disease who wanders off the unit periodically. The problem is discussed in conference and the instructor decides that since the approaches that have been used have not been successful, brainstorming for new ideas is in order. The teacher explains that the students are to spend 5 minutes writing down any possible ways that the patient's wandering could be controlled. After the 5 minutes are up, all the students share their ideas, and combinations and revisions of ideas are formulated. A few of the many ideas that the instructor might record are:

1. Reorient the patient every 10 minutes.
2. Lock the doors to the unit.
3. Put an identification sign on the patient in case she gets lost.
4. Place a child's gate across the doorway to the patient's room to prevent her from getting out.
5. Have the patient wear bells on her ankles so nurses can hear where she is walking.

The group would spend a few minutes weighing the ideas for safety, practicality, impact on patient dignity, effect on other patients, time required, and cost. Final solutions would then be formulated and tested.

Although the brainstorming technique is used on a limited basis in nursing education, its potential value is great, and it is a useful addition to a teacher's repertoire of skills.

Debate

Debate as a teaching strategy has lost popularity over the past few decades, yet its use has never completely died out and has made a comeback of sorts in the last few years. The debate method is a reasonable choice for educators who are preparing nurses and future nurses to take a stand on professional issues.

Although debate is a form of discussion, it differs pointedly from general discussion. Whereas discussion is based on open-mindedness and involves searching for solutions and compromise, debate is based on the belief that someone has found a solution and has only to convince others of its rightness. Discussion is basically cooperative, while debate is competitive (Hoover, 1965).

Debate involves a series of timed speeches for and against a specific question or proposal. This process actually serves several purposes: It reinforces research and oral communication skills, helps students learn organization of material and logical thought patterns, and fosters critical and divergent thinking (Jackson, 1973).

Nurses often have to defend their professional beliefs and practices. They are sometimes placed in adversarial positions and frequently have to resolve conflicts. Learning how to prepare evidence and rational positions and to build irrefutable arguments is an invaluable experience for nursing students.

Techniques of Debate

The issue to be debated is worded as either a "Resolved" statement or a question. For example, a debate issue could be stated as "Resolved, that a 6-month preceptorship should be made available to all new graduates beginning their first job" or "Should specialist nurses be required to float to hospital units outside of their specialty?"

Hoover suggests that three questions should be answered in the course of a debate: "(1) Is there a need? (2) Will the specific plan of the affirmative remedy the existing state of affairs? and (3) Is the plan feasible or desirable?" (1965; 233). The affirmative team answers these questions positively, and the negative team, if possible, refutes them and supports the status quo.

For every debate, there should be two learners who will argue affirmatively and two negatively. Students may select the topics or be assigned to them, and they may or may not be permitted to select the groups with which they work.

Time limits should be made explicit when the assignment is given. Usually the first constructive speeches are limited to 5 to 10 minutes each, and the rebuttal speeches, 3 to 5 minutes. The instructor should plan for time at the end of the debate for general class discussion; the amount will be determined by the topic and by the available class time.

The organization of the debate usually follows this format: first affirmative speaker, first negative speaker, second affirmative speaker, second negative speaker. Following these four constructive speeches are the rebuttal speeches in this order: first negative speaker, first affirmative speaker, second negative speaker, second affirmative speaker. The two speakers on each side decide how to divide their information in a logical way. It may be possible, for instance, for the first affirmative speaker to establish the need for the resolution and the second to explain the steps of the plan and its feasibility. When all eight speeches have been given, the audience enters the debate.

The teacher usually instructs the audience before the debate to make a brief list of the opposing arguments and to jot down notes for future questions. When the time arrives for audience discussion, students have the opportunity to question the debaters and to provide additional arguments on either side. The role of the teacher at this time is that of discussion leader.

The last step in the process is evaluating the debate. Some debates, especially those under the aegis of debating clubs, are formally evaluated by a panel of judges who decide which side has won. In nursing education it seems unnecessary and perhaps undesirable to declare a winner in the debate. Rather, each side should be evaluated in terms of the soundness and effectiveness of its arguments, the clarity of its communication, and defense of its position. The audience as well as the teacher may write an evaluation on these points. Having to write a detailed evaluation also serves to keep the audience attentive during the debate.

Debating not only achieves many educational objectives but can be exciting and fun for students once they have recovered from their fright at the idea of being "on stage." If the instructor works closely with students to help them prepare, the entire experience should be a positive one for the class.

Advantages and Disadvantages of Debate

An advantage of the debate strategy is that it expands students' perspectives on given issues, perhaps creating doubt about or providing further evidence to support previously held views. Debate helps students develop the technique of persuasion and reduces their awkwardness in defending controversial issues. In debate, students work together as partners. This collaboration can be a positive experience as students learn how to work in a dyadic relationship, capitalizing on each other's strengths. It also provides students with a wider forum for their efforts than a written paper does and may give them a greater sense of achievement. Finally, in the process of rebuttal students learn to listen carefully and to analyze quickly what is being said so that they can give a logical refutation.

Disadvantages of the debate method are relatively few. Some people criticize debate for fostering a false view of issues as being either black or white; they suggest that education should focus on cooperation rather than divergence and arguments (Hoover, 1965). The biggest practical disadvantage is that some students may have to defend a position to which they are not committed.

Summary of Research

Osborn's initial research revealed that engineers produced 44% more worthwhile ideas when brainstorming as a group than when they worked alone (Collaros & Anderson, 1969). DeCecco (1968) summarized research done on brainstorming in the early 1960s. He found evidence that creative problem solving increases with training in brainstorming, that "more good ideas are produced with brainstorming than with conventional techniques" (p. 460), and that students who took courses that included brainstorming along with other creative problem-solving methods obtained higher scores on creative ability than students who did not take such courses. These early findings provide some evidence of the potential worth of brainstorming as a means of increasing creativity and effective problem solving.

Some other researchers investigated the conditions under which brainstorming should be applied. Joelson and Eliseo (1961) found support for Osborn's first rule that criticism of ideas should wait until all ideas have been generated. These researchers found that groups of students who did not critique their ideas produced greater numbers and a higher quality of ideas than groups who concurrently evaluated their ideas. Collaros and Anderson (1969) discovered that the creativity of members of brainstorming groups was inhibited when members felt that experts in the group might disapprove of some of the ideas.

Three research groups reported results conflicting with Osborn's finding that group brainstorming is superior to individual work. These more recent studies revealed that the most effective brainstorming takes place when individuals first work on their own and then pool their ideas (Bouchard & Hare, 1970; Madsen & Finger, 1978; Maginn & Harris, 1980). It is thought that group productivity may be limited by factors such as fear of nonverbal criticism, domination by some group members, and the whole group getting side-tracked.

Additional investigation into brainstorming might yield worthwhile results. Some of the conflicting reports invite further study. Is individual brainstorming the best route to follow? Does this technique really foster creativity, and if so, in what settings and situations? If students are taught via brainstorming, do they use the method later in their professional practice?

Little substantive research has been done on the methodology of seminar and debate, perhaps because these techniques are used less frequently than others or are used only in highly selective situations. It would be useful for teachers to know, however, which learning situations are most appropriate for these techniques and how they can be implemented to yield the desired learning outcomes. Does the seminar method help develop group leadership abilities? Do either seminars or debates contribute to the development of critical thinking? Are the learning outcomes for debate any different when formal debate rather than informal debate is used? Does the competition in debate enhance or impede learning?

All of these questions could lead to productive research efforts.

References

Anderson NE: The use of the seminar as a teaching technique with senior undergraduate nursing students. *J Nurs Educ* (Feb) 1980; 19:20–25.

Bouchard TJ, Hare M: Size, performance, and potential in brainstorming groups. *J Applied Psych* 1970; 54:51–55.

Collaros PA, Anderson LR: Effect of perceived expertness upon creativity of members of brainstorming groups. *J Applied Psych* 1969; 53:159–163.

Cooper SS: Methods of teaching revisited: formal discussion: the seminar. *J Contin Educ Nurs* (May/June) 1979; 10:39–40.

DeCecco JP: *The Psychology of Learning and Instruction.* Prentice-Hall, 1968.

Hoover KH: The debate: valid teaching method? *Clearing House* 1965; 40:232–235.

Jackson M: Debate: a neglected teaching tool. *Peabody J of Educ* 1973; 50:150–154.

Joelson EW, Eliseo TS: An experimental study of the effectiveness of brainstorming. *J Applied Psych* 1961; 45:45–49.

Madsen DB, Finger JR: Comparison of a written feedback procedure, group brainstorming, and individual brainstorming. *J Applied Psych* 1978; 63:120–123.

Maginn BK, Harris RJ: Effects of anticipated evaluation on individual
   brainstorming performance. *J Applied Psych* 1980; 65:219–225.
Osborn AF: *Applied Imagination.* Scribner's, 1957.
Vande Zande GA: The use of the seminar to teach group process and
   group leadership with registered nurse students at the baccalaureate
   level. *J Nurs Educ* 1987; 26:37–38.

Chapter 6

Individualized Learning

Nursing faculty talk a lot about the importance of meeting the individual learning needs of students, but other than in clinical settings they are usually more involved in standardization than individualization. How can teachers meet individual student needs when there are 30 or more students in a class and when there is so much information to be taught? Indeed, it is an impossible task unless the teacher departs from traditional methods and traditional classroom structure and tries a program of individualized or self-paced learning.

It takes a leap of faith for many faculty who have never personally experienced individualized learning packages to try this approach. The teacher who has not previously been exposed to this form of teaching or learning may view it skeptically at first. Is it a sound educational method? Isn't it just an easy way out for a lazy teacher? Doesn't the teacher lose a lot of control of the learning process? Won't many students do as little work as possible just to get by? Isn't the expertise of the teacher wasted? Experience and research have demonstrated that individualized learning programs can be as sound educationally as any other and that they have no more pitfalls than any of the more traditional ways of teaching.

For the teacher who is concerned about tailoring instruction to individual needs or who is faced with the unenviable task of teaching learners from different educational and social backgrounds, individualized learning may be just the thing. This approach probably is best suited to experienced teachers who have already taught the course by traditional methods.

Although some nursing programs have implemented self-learning packages or modules for their entire curriculum, more have used them for only some courses or parts of courses. Using individualized learning for whole versus parts of curricula has both advantages and disadvantages, which you will see as we go along.

History of Individualized Learning

Individualized learning programs were first developed in the 1960s by educators who wanted to place more emphasis on student learning than on the process of teaching. They wanted a means of helping more students succeed at learning, and they wanted students to be more actively involved in the learning process. They emphasized the principles of behavioral psychology, with its stress on positive reinforcement for learning. In these years several psychologists and educators developed programs that have been further refined and are still used today.

Fred Keller of Arizona State University first developed the personalized system of instruction (PSI), sometimes referred to as the Keller plan. Keller (1968) delineated five components of his method that set it apart from conventional teaching methods:

1. *Self-pacing.* The student progresses through the course at a comfortable speed that fits his or her learning style and life-style.

2. *Content mastery.* The student can move on to new content only after mastering previous content.

3. *Lectures and demonstrations as motivation.* The student can attend these optional events only after certain material has been mastered, and they are not tested on the material.

4. *Stress on the written word.* The student is given most of the content of the course in written form and thus retains more control over the learning process.

5. *Use of proctors.* Teaching aides are available to give immediate feedback on unit tests and to prescribe individualized remedial work.

In PSI, students are given a series of written assignments that cover various learning units in a course. They are also given reading and laboratory assignments to complete at their own pace. They are encouraged (but not required) to do the assignments during scheduled class time because proctors are available to answer questions. The written assignments may be from a standard textbook, a programmed text, or other printed materials. A list of study questions is also included to guide the students' reading and study. When the student feels prepared, he or she goes to class to take a readiness test. If he or she passes, the next assignment is given and the student is eligible to attend the first lecture or demonstration. If the student has not mastered the content, the proctor suggests some additional study activities. There is a final examination in the course, which the student is expected to take before the end of the semester. Incomplete grades are given only in special cases.

Concurrently in the 1960s, Samuel Postlethwait of Purdue University was developing his audio-tutorial system of learning (Postlethwait, Novak & Murray, 1972). This program differs from Keller's PSI primarily in the use of audiotapes and other audiovisuals rather than written materials and in the use of mandatory group sessions.

The audio-tutorial system is implemented in a campus learning center. Students conduct independent study sessions at booths equipped with a tape recorder, a movie projector, and any other materials needed for the week's lessons. Each student is given a set of behavioral objectives for the week, a printed study guide, and a textbook. The student receives detailed instructions and guidance for the lesson through the audiotapes made by the professor. If the student can achieve the behavioral objectives before beginning the lesson, he or she need not progress with the rest of the week's work. But all students, by means of spending as much time as necessary during the week, must accomplish all of the objectives.

At the end of the week, students attend a large general assembly session led by the senior instructor. This time is used to lecture on required information, provide guest lecturers, show long films, conduct help sessions, and give major exams. Following the large assembly, small assembly sessions of eight students are held for 45 minutes to quiz students orally and in writing.

Less self-pacing occurs with the audio-tutorial system since a unit must be completed each week. However, within the week students can schedule study time to suit themselves, and they can take as little or as much time as they need to achieve the objectives. The use of audiovisuals as well as printed materials is advantageous for adaptations to individual learning styles.

Since the 1960s several other variations on individualized learning have appeared. The process has come to be associated with many terms, including self-paced instruction, autotutorial instruction, teaching-learning units, learning modules, learning activity packages, and individualized study packages, to name a few.

Individualized Learning Modules

The systems of individualized instruction described by Cardarelli (1972), Layton (1975), and Thompson (1978) are all outgrowths of the vanguard projects in the 1960s. These authors describe the use of learning activity packages or learning modules as they are still being widely used today.

Module Components

Almost all individualized learning modules (as I will refer to them) have the following components:

single concept topic

behavioral objectives

pretest

learning activities

self-evaluations

posttest

The topic for a module is a single concept. If you were teaching a course in medical-surgical nursing that incorporated problems of digestion, metabolism, endocrine function, and elimination, you would have at least four modules and very likely more. For instance, the concept of elimination could be taught in one module, but it would be more effective to develop two modules, one for intestinal elimination and one for urinary elimination.

Behavioral objectives in a module are no different from those you have already learned about and written. They express, in clear language, what the student will be able to do on completion of the module. These objectives need to be quite specific so that both student and teacher know what is expected and whether it has been achieved by the end of the module.

A pretest is usually but not always included in a module. If the teacher is sure that no student would be familiar with any of the information in the module, a pretest is not needed. If, for example, the concept of the module is the history of nursing and all the students are 18-year-old college freshmen, it would be reasonable to assume that all would be encountering this information for the first time.

Most modules written for nursing curricula do include a pretest, for two reasons. First, nursing students today come from heterogeneous backgrounds. A class may consist of many 18- to 20-year-olds who entered college right after high school, but it will also include second degree students, transfer students, and people who have entered college after working at some other job for a period of time. Some of these enrollees may already know some of the information in the module. A second reason for including a pretest is that students learn different information as they move through a nursing curriculum. Although the basic curriculum is standardized, students have differing clinical experiences, carry out different projects, and may take a variety of elective courses. A student may be familiar with some parts of the module because of these experiences. RN learners certainly come to a class with varying experiences that must be taken into account.

The instructor may look at the pretest results, but usually they are for student use only. The pretest helps students evaluate which sections of the module they might skip over and which ones they need to study from the bottom up. One other feature sometimes seen in pretests is a section that evaluates prerequisite knowledge. Thus, if a student performs poorly on the questions about previously learned material, he or she would be instructed to review this material before proceeding.

Learning activities make up the most creative portion of the module for the teacher. Contrary to the prototypes of Keller and Postlethwait, modules today usually encompass a much wider variety of learning activities that enable students to learn in their preferred modes. Written materials such as textbooks, information sheets, written lectures or speeches, pamphlets and books from voluntary agencies or private companies, study questions, programmed instruction, and diagrams are all appropriate for learning modules. Audiovisual materials are often included, as are computer programs or games. Students may also be asked to practice laboratory skills, make community visits, participate in discussion groups, or give presentations. Attendance at some lectures or seminars may be required or optional. If clinical practice is part of the module, specific clinical activities are designated.

If possible, students are given alternative activities that will help them meet the same objectives. If the same information is available in a textbook and on a filmstrip, students may be told to use one or the other, depending on their preferences.

Students have access to a faculty member or teaching assistant during the time they are involved in learning activities. Someone may be available during scheduled class times or during additional office hours. There may be scheduled group discussions during which students are encouraged to ask questions about the material they are studying and faculty members can assess student progress informally.

While students are participating in learning activities, they should be checking back occasionally to see whether they are working toward the objectives. One way for them to assess how well they are achieving the objectives is for them to use self-evaluation tools. A self-test is usually included at the end of every lesson or subconcept. It is generally some form of short quiz. If the student does not achieve a perfect score on the self-test, he or she must reenter the module for the appropriate lesson.

Posttests are used to determine whether students have mastered module objectives. The posttest may be a written quiz or examination, a written assignment such as a nursing care plan, a live or videotaped skill demonstration, or a demonstration of clinical performance. If the student's performance on the posttest indicates mastery of the objectives, he or she can move on to the next module or course of study. Failure to demonstrate mastery results in the student having to repeat appropriate learning activities or being given alternative activities to meet his or her particular needs.

Grading Mastery Learning

Most individualized learning packages are grounded in the principle of mastery learning, or competency-based learning. That is, the student continues to engage in learning activities until the material is mastered (usually considered 80%–100% performance level) or until competence can be demonstrated. Grading systems in individualized learning programs vary. Some programs are so committed to mastery learning that every student is given an almost indefinite period of time to achieve mastery. In such a system, most students earn A's in the course, and some students may receive Incomplete or Withdrawal grades. The only case for failure is if the student cannot achieve mastery by the final deadline, whether that is at the end of the semester or the end of the candidacy period in the school. A grading system in which almost all students get A's may be unacceptable to many institutions because it gives an image of grade inflation.

In variations of mastery learning, a variety of grade levels can be assigned. For example, students can contract for a grade of A, B, or C. If they master objectives (or modules) 1–4, they may get a C. If they complete objective/module 5 they obtain a B, and completing objective/module 6 may earn an A. Objectives/modules 5 and 6 in this system would have to represent more than the minimum level of acceptable behavior. These additional objectives or modules may represent a greater depth of understanding and application of the information learned in objectives/modules 1–4, or they may include additional information that is not needed for minimal competency but that provides enrichment. In nursing programs where some courses are taught by individualized learning and others are not, this more traditional type of grading system may be more acceptable than that in a pure mastery system.

Time limits can also be imposed in some of the hybrid forms of mastery learning. In Postlethwait's audio-tutorial system, each learning unit had to be completed within 1 week. In some courses of this type, if the student does not complete the first few units on time, he or she must withdraw from the course. Schiller and Markle (1978) describe the use of "doomsday contingencies" in which an instructor requires students to meet certain deadlines within the course or else meet with the instructor before being allowed to go on. Failure to meet further deadlines results in a failing grade.

These variations on mastery learning reflect the restrictions placed on some faculty who work within a relatively inflexible academic system in which deadlines must be met and grading systems adhered to. Such restrictions do not preclude the use of individualized learning modules, but they do necessitate adjustments in implementation.

Developing a Module

Plans for developing a module should be undertaken weeks or months before it will be needed, because module development is a time-consuming process.

Content   Planning begins with consideration of the content of the module. If you have already taught the course by traditional methods, this step will involve looking at the established content and dividing it into logical conceptual units. It may be helpful to follow the outline of the textbook that you plan to require for the course.

Let's imagine that you want to develop a module for the topic of intestinal elimination. In your previous teaching of this course material and in accordance with the textbook, you decide that the important content will revolve around assessment of intestinal elimination, infectious and inflammatory disorders, and obstructive disorders, with accompanying nursing care.

Behavioral Objectives The second step in the development process is formulating behavioral objectives for the module. With due deliberation, you arrive at the following objectives:

1. Perform an assessment of intestinal elimination on a live simulated patient (videotaped or performed during a scheduled laboratory session), correctly including all critical elements.

2. Explain the effects of infection and inflammation on the gastrointestinal tract.

3. Differentiate between any three infectious or inflammatory gastrointestinal disorders in terms of pathology, patient problems, and nursing interventions.

4. View a filmstrip simulation on constipation and diarrhea and list the patient's problems, your proposed interventions, and rationale for those interventions.

5. Analyze why a given list of nursing interventions would be used for a patient with an obstructed small bowel.

6. Evaluate the nursing care delivered by a nurse (on videotape) who is caring for a patient who has had surgery for an incarcerated inguinal hernia.

7. Write and implement (on videotape) a teaching plan for a patient with a selected inflammatory disorder.

Learning Activities You now have a pretty good idea of where you want the student to go, but you still have to decide how you are going to help the student get there. So, you plan the content and the learning activities. Choose a variety of learning activities that would be appropriate for different learning style preferences, cognitive styles, and student response styles (see Chapter 3). For example, some learning activities should stress abstractions, some should focus on concrete information; some should be visual, some auditory, some tactile. Activities ought to be balanced between those that can be accomplished alone and those that two students or more could work on. Some activities could be competitive and some, collaborative. Keep in mind the amount of time that the student will have to complete the module and the learning resources that are available.

The first unit in our sample module deals with assessment of intestinal elimination, and the first objective explains the outcome behavior. You arrive at the following learning activities:

Unit I

1. Read pages 216 to 222 in your textbook in light of the study questions on Handout #1.

2. Select one of the following activities:
    a. View filmstrip #36, "Assessment of Intestinal Function."
    b. Listen to audiotape #51, "Step-by-Step History Taking and Physical Assessment, Part 5."

3. Practice doing an assessment of intestinal elimination.

All of the materials needed to complete these activities should be readily available to the student. Any written materials should be included in the module packet or should be in the school library. Audiovisuals and equipment for a practice lab ought to be accessible in a centralized location. Students should not have to waste time searching for learning materials. Subsequent units to meet the rest of the objectives would be developed in a similar manner.

Pretest   Now it is time to backtrack a little. You have identified content and learning activities. At this point you can determine whether you need a pretest, and if so, what will go into it. Because this course is offered in the junior year, students may come to it with varying preparation, so a pretest is in order.

Part of the pretest should include questions about normal anatomy and physiology of intestinal elimination, as this is important prerequisite material. Directions that accompany the pretest should specify that if the anatomy and physiology questions are answered incorrectly, the student should review that information in an appropriate textbook. If the pretest reveals mastery of certain units of content, the student should be informed that he or she may skip that part of the module.

If you want the student to do a self-evaluation and receive instant feedback, place the answers to the pretest at the end of the module. If you wish to see the pretests and use them as a source of individual student guidance, you can grade them and meet with the students to discuss the results.

Self-evaluation Self-evaluation guides should be developed to accompany each unit. These guides are short quizzes, based on the objectives, that enable the students to check their progress. The answers to the self-evaluation guides should be placed at the end of the module for quick student feedback. Students need to know what level of performance constitutes mastery of the unit (usually 80%–100%). Less-than-acceptable performance means that the student must go back into the unit and repeat the appropriate learning activities.

You can also design the process so that at the end of the page with the self-evaluation answers are additional activities to be used if mastery has not been accomplished.

Posttest and Grading While you are writing self-evaluation test questions, take time to develop the posttest. The posttest is usually, at least in part, a written examination. Some of the objectives will be measured in this way by means of multiple-choice and matching items, essay questions, and so on. Actually, you should devise two or three forms of the written posttest. It is not an easy task to write two, let alone three, roughly equivalent exams, but it is necessary in the case of mastery learning. If a student fails the first posttest, he or she must go back to the learning activities and then has an opportunity to retake the posttest. Obviously, it is not a good idea to give the same test again in a short period of time, so an equivalent form is needed. If students are allowed a third retake, a third form of the examination should be available. Remember that all forms of the exam must be derived from the objectives, not just from the content. If many students are failing the second exam, and certainly if they fail the third, you should examine the tests and the learning activities to find out where the problem lies.

Students should be permitted to take the posttest whenever they are ready to do so, and they should get feedback as soon as possible. If you are not regularly available for giving posttests, perhaps you can arrange for a secretary or teaching assistant to administer them. Grading should be done within a day or two so that students who have failed can begin remedial activities.

If you refer back to the objectives for your module on intestinal elimination, you will see that more than just a written posttest is indicated in order to measure achievement of the objectives. Students also have to perform a skill demonstration in person or on video and write a teaching plan and implement it on videotape. These assignments have to be satisfactorily completed before moving on to the next module. The last three objectives involve writing a nursing care plan and analyzing and evaluating nursing interventions. These objectives could be measured by written papers to be handed in at any time or could be a part of the written posttest.

Just another note about grading. In our example, if a student mastered the seven objectives, he or she would receive a "Pass" for the module. If there were five modules in your entire course and all five were mastered, the student would receive a "Pass" or an A grade, depending on the system in your institution. Tiered grading could also be built in by working on the assumption that five of the seven objectives listed (1–5) represent the minimal level of learning for the module and when mastered will result in a grade of C. If the student wished to achieve a B grade, he or she would also have to master objectives 6 and 7.

Students with the motivation and time might choose to work on an additional objective, mastery of which would yield an A for the module. You could be creative in deciding what this type of enrichment objective might be. Perhaps it would be something like "Write a four-page paper on cultural influences on bowel elimination habits and beliefs" or "Interview a gerontological nurse specialist regarding elimination problems and corresponding interventions for elderly institutionalized people."

With this system, the course grade would be an average of the five module grades. You could also design the course so that completion of the five modules would result in a grade of B. Students who wished to earn an A would have to complete a sixth enrichment module. There are many avenues for creativity in designing modules and constructing courses of individualized learning.

Introductory Material   Every module, but especially the first in a series, should be accompanied by an introductory page that explains the overall approach and procedures. It should include instructions on how to work through the module, how to use the pretest and self-evaluation guides, what procedures to use for handing in assignments and scheduling tests, how grades will be determined, and what the roles of the student and teacher are.

Here is a prototype for such an introduction:

This packet represents the first in a series of five modules that will guide your learning in this course. The course being 15 weeks in length, you can see that you will have approximately 3 weeks to complete each module, if you want to spread the work out evenly. However, you may move at your own pace and take the posttest whenever you have completed the module. You must successfully complete module #1 before progressing to module #2, and so on.

Read the objectives of the module carefully before beginning any activities and refer back to them frequently. All learning experiences and evaluations will be based on the objectives. After reading the objectives, take the pretest. The answers to the pretest are found at the back of the packet (but no peeking ahead of time allowed!). You can find out immediately after taking the test how little or how much you know about the content in the module. The pretest is divided into units that correspond to the units of the module. If you get all the answers to any of the units correct, it is your option to skip the learning activities of that unit and just take the posttest.

All of the learning activity materials are either in your packet, in your textbook, in the school library, or in the Learning Laboratory; each learning activity section will indicate where to find materials. We will have a discussion group during scheduled class hour every Thursday. You should attend at least 7 of the 14 discussions, unless you make other individual arrangements with me. The topics for the discussion will be posted 2 weeks in advance. You should come prepared to intelligently discuss the topic (which is based on the modules) and to ask questions about any material that may be puzzling you or for which you want clarification.

When you have successfully completed the self-evaluation guides for each module and handed in any required assignments, you may schedule a posttest with me. I am always available to give posttests during scheduled class hours, usually during my office hours, and at other times by appointment. Some posttests I will grade immediately. For others, I will have your grades within 24 hours. If you receive less than 80% on the written posttest, you must take the test again after completing some remedial work.

Your grade for the course will be calculated as explained on the next page. In keeping with college policy, a grade of Incomplete can be granted only in cases of hard-

ship such as prolonged illness. If you do not complete all
five modules by the last day of the course, therefore, you
will receive an F grade. Please budget your time carefully.

Although you may go over this type of information during the
first class session, it should also be in writing so that the students
have it to refer to throughout the semester.

Evaluating the Module

When you have completed your initial work on the module, you
should pilot test it. If you can do so, have at least five students of
varying ability try each module so that you can find any flaws or
snags before you put the module to actual use. You might find that
some of the directions are unclear, that some activities are too time
consuming or too difficult, or that a greater variety of learning
activities is needed.

After the module is used for the first time in the actual course,
you should have the students write a brief evaluation of the process. Some things may still need to be changed if all students are
progressing at the same rate through the modules, if slow learners
are not improving even with remedial activities, if too many students need to take the posttest more than once, or if no students
take advantage of enrichment activities (Clark, 1978).

Commercial modules are available from some nursing textbook publishers. If you do not have the time or feel you lack the
expertise to develop a module, you might be wise to investigate
this option. Evaluation of commercially prepared modules is also
important to see how well they meet your needs and how well they
fit into the school setting.

Uses of Individualized Learning

Individualized, self-paced learning has been used in just about all
educational settings. It has been used in baccalaureate and associate degree nursing programs for the purpose of teaching basic
skills, physical assessment, medical-surgical, and parent-child nursing courses. It has also been used quite successfully in health care
agencies for continuing education programs (Craig, 1982; Gentine,
1980; Hinthorne, 1980; Rufo, 1985). In addition, many graduate
programs have based some of their courses on this method of
learning (Chinn & Hunt, 1975).

The programs for which learning modules have been a real boon are those that enroll primarily nontraditional students. Both mobility curricula that prepare licensed practical nurses to become registered nurses and upper-division baccalaureate nursing programs for registered nurses can benefit from this form of instruction, which enables students to learn what they need to learn and move quickly past that which they already know. Nontraditional students may be less resentful of having to repeat courses they've already had if they are allowed to learn in this manner.

Roles of the Student and Teacher

When individualized learning is used, the role of the student changes dramatically. Instead of being relatively or completely passive in learning, the student becomes totally active. He or she cannot sit in the back of the classroom and daydream or even quietly listen while the teacher does most of the work. Rather, the student must be studying, manipulating information, preparing for discussions, and probably taking many more tests of one type or another.

The student now has to take on a large part of the responsibility for his or her own education, and that can be frightening at first. Until students realize that their learning is still being closely guided by the faculty member, they may even feel resentful at being on their own and having to shoulder so much of the responsibility. Once they are used to the system, attitudes improve.

Student attitudes toward individualized learning have been explored by many researchers. The findings indicate that students like the method at least as well as traditional strategies when they become accustomed to it—in fact, they usually prefer it (Baskin, 1962; Kulik, Kulik & Cohen, 1979; Mueller, 1974; Ostrow, 1986; Shavelson & Munger, 1970; Thompson, 1972). In a study of baccalaureate nursing students, Stein et al (1972) found favorable attitudes but also found that students wanted deadlines to work toward, rather than having to set their own time limits. Fisher and MacWhinney (1976), in their review of 89 studies conducted between 1962 and 1975, deduced that what students liked most about individualized learning were the freedom, stimulation, ease of learning, and fact that they felt they learned more.

To provide evidence that favorable attitudes toward PSI were not just the result of a novelty effect, Linder and Whitehurst (1973) correlated attitudes toward PSI with the number of PSI courses taken. They found no correlation but rather discovered that PSI received consistently high ratings, regardless of how many courses students had taken.

The student's role in individualized instruction is to choose the appropriate learning activities and use them to master the content—to achieve the objectives. Organizing and distributing study time is an inherent—and for some students, the most difficult—part of that role. Compulsive students may drive themselves relentlessly to move through the modules as quickly as possible. Procrastinators may only be motivated by doomsday contingencies. Yet, time management is an important part of the learning process.

The teacher by no means abdicates all responsibility once the course begins. Instructors of modular courses do not go to the South Seas following the pretest only to return the last day of the course. Rather, they are involved throughout the course in monitoring student progress, leading group discussions or other class meetings, grading examinations and other assignments, and designing remedial programs for students who are having problems.

It is true that the teacher may not be as busy during the semester as colleagues who are teaching a conventional course, but remember that many hours of preparation go into designing, testing, and revising the modules before the course begins. In the end the workload probably evens out.

The significant role change for the instructor is moving from disseminator of information to facilitator of learning. The teacher guides and supports the student in his or her individual quest for learning. The teacher's role has evolved from that of performer to that of diagnostician, planner, and prescriber. Not all teachers are comfortable in or happy with this kind of role, but many find it exciting.

Advantages and Disadvantages of Individualized Learning

The modular learning technique has advantages for both students and teachers.

Students benefit by learning to be independent and by learning to rely less on the teacher as the sole source of information and more on their own abilities to find the answers to questions and the solutions to problems. The potential exists for students to develop and gain confidence in their critical thinking and analysis abilities. The built-in feedback feature and the mastery principle of the modules can shore up students' self-esteem and provide them with much more reward and success than they have experienced before. The success in learning can help to build motivation for future learning as well. The individualization aspect of this teaching method is one of its greatest advantages. Students can learn in their preferred styles and study at times that mesh with their lifestyles and biological rhythms. They can work at their own pace, within certain restraints. Bright students need not be held back in their search for knowledge, and weaker students can take the time they need to learn the body of knowledge.

For teachers the benefits may not be as obvious, but they are there. Instructors who are frustrated by not having the time to help students who are struggling with the course material in the traditional system have that opportunity in the individualized approach. They can better diagnose learning difficulties and help students correct them. Teachers are also freed from having to repeat the same material year after year, which can become monotonous. The opportunities for creativity in designing modules and conducting small discussion groups can lend new interest to teaching.

Evaluation of the entire learning process is augmented by the modular approach to teaching. Because the teacher is not as involved in preparation for and conduct of daily classes, he or she has the time to look at the learning process objectively. Pretest results can be analyzed. Meetings can be scheduled with students to assess their progress. Posttests can be closely scrutinized to determine common problem areas. All this information can be used to help students through the course and to revise modules for future use.

Finally, individualized learning packages make it possible for a curriculum to be standardized, if that is desired. All students taking any section of a course should achieve comparable learning if they are all using the same package and are subjected to the same objectives and learning activities. The modules can hold the curriculum constant in spite of changes in the composition of the faculty from year to year.

As always, disadvantages go hand in hand with the benefits. Students who have never before experienced this kind of independence in learning may flounder at first. They may procrastinate and, if not guided, may fall so far behind that catching up becomes impossible. Students may also feel that this method is too impersonal; they may prefer traditional classrooms where they have daily contact with the professor.

Research has revealed that students sometimes feel overworked in a modular learning system. Faculty get so enthusiastic about designing learning activities and measurement techniques for the modules that they don't realize how much is being required of students. The requirements for one module may seem as extensive as those for an entire course. Pilot testing of the modules can give the teacher a realistic idea of how much time each module should take.

In the face of claims that individualized instruction saves learning or study time, researchers have compared the amount of time it takes to learn a body of material by traditional versus individualized methods. The conclusions to be drawn are unclear. Born and Davis (1974) found that students in a university psychology class spent slightly more study time when using PSI. Nursing students learning with a CPR module took less study time than those taught by lecture/demonstration (Friesen & Stotts, 1984). In a meta-analysis of 72 studies, researchers reported 4 studies that found equal study time (Kulik, Kulik & Cohen, 1979).

Researchers have also investigated possible correlations between the amount of time devoted to studying a module and achievement on a posttest. If individualized instruction is fulfilling its destiny of allowing students of varying ability and learning styles to study as much as they need to in order to learn the material, there should be no relationship between study time and achievement. Two nursing studies demonstrated this lack of correlation (Koniak, 1985; Osborn & Thompson, 1976). Fisher and MacWhinney (1976) discovered three studies concluding no correlation and seven showing a positive correlation.

Individualized learning can present some problems for instructors, too. As already mentioned, it takes a tremendous amount of time to prepare the modules before a course begins. Teachers may not have this kind of lead time or may feel that they are not being compensated for it. Modules need frequent revisions and updating, which are also time consuming.

As students move through the modules at their own rate of speed, it is possible to have one class of students working on several different modules at any one time. This situation can present problems in accompanying clinical courses. For example, if you have a clinical group of ten students, three of whom are learning the bowel elimination module, four studying the module on digestion, and four progressed to the module on endocrine disorders, you might have difficulty finding appropriate clinical assignments. Even more problematic is finding commonalities to discuss in post-conferences so that all students can benefit from the content.

Research on Individualized Learning

A great deal of research has been conducted on individualized learning in the last two and a half decades. The main variables of interest have been amount of learning, long-term retention of knowledge, attitudes toward the method, and amount and effects of study time.

Most of the studies have focused on a comparison of results between classes taught by traditional methods (lecture/discussion) and those taught by PSI, autotutorial, or modular methods of some variety. By far the majority of researchers have compared the means of final exam grades, although some have compared results on skill attainment. In 1962, for example, Baskin summarized the results of a 4-year experiment at Antioch College; using several types of written posttests, both control and experimental groups consistently demonstrated equivalent learning.

Shavelson and Munger (1970) found that for a high school science course a group using individualized, self-paced learning did significantly better on the posttest than a group learning by traditional methods.

Born, Gledhill and Davis (1972) taught psychology to 60 university students using either the PSI or lecture/discussion methods and found no differences in scores on multiple-choice questions, but the PSI group did significantly better on fill-in and essay questions. This is not surprising since students in modular courses often get more practice in writing.

Also in 1972, Stein et al compared the results for 60 baccalaureate nursing students who were taught by the two methods and discovered no differences either in final examination scores or in clinical performance. Friesen and Stotts reported similar results in teaching cardiopulmonary resuscitation in 1984.

Two more nursing studies, one by Myers and Greenwood in 1978 and another by Koniak in 1985, revealed autotutorial modules to be superior to lecture/discussion when written exams were given.

In 1974 Mueller, in an educational measurement class, found

the same level of learning in groups taught by both methods, but in the same year Born and Davis discovered that their students in the PSI section of a psychology class had superior performance over the traditional section.

Three published reports of research summaries or meta-analyses also found mixed results. Most studies reported that individualized learning groups performed better on posttests than traditionally taught groups, many found no significant difference between the groups, and a very few documented superior performance by the traditional groups (Fisher & MacWhinney, 1976; Kulik, Kulik & Cohen, 1979; Mintzes, 1975).

It is clear then that individualized instruction is at least as good as or better than lecture/discussion for short-term learning. It is possible, of course, that the Hawthorne effect could be operating in many of the studies, especially those conducted the first time students were exposed to the modular approach.

Long-term retention of knowledge has been studied by fewer researchers. Three studies that compared individualized to traditional methods revealed no differences in retention of learning. Baskin (1962) studied retention after two years; Thompson (1972) looked at results of a National League for Nursing exam given a year after a course; Pensivy (1977) used results of nursing state board examinations. Kulik, Kulik and Cohen (1979) found eight studies in which delayed retention was superior when PSI was used.

Although the research evidence related to individualized instruction, as in many educational arenas, is by no means conclusive, it does provide substantial support for the method's usefulness and dependability as a teaching strategy. Inquiry into this methodology should continue. Is there an ideal format for module design? Does module length affect learning? Do students perform better or progress more smoothly when time constraints are built into the modules? Is there an interaction effect between student age/maturity and amount or ease of learning with the individualized approach? Many such questions remain unanswered and provide a fertile field for future study.

References

Baskin S: Experiment in independent study. *J Exper Educ* 1962; 31:183–185.
Born DG, Davis ML: Amount and distribution of study in a personalized

instruction course and in a lecture course. *J Applied Behavior Analysis* 1974; 7:365–375.

Born DG, Gledhill SM, Davis ML: Examination performance in lecture-discussion and personalized instruction courses. *J Applied Behavior Analysis* 1972; 5:33–43.

Cardarelli SM: The LAP—A feasible vehicle of individualization. *Educ Tech* (March) 1972; 12:23–29.

Chinn PL, Hunt VO: Modules in child nursing instruction. *Nurs Outlook* 1975; 23:650–653.

Clark CC: *Classroom Skills for Nurse Educators.* Springer, 1978.

Craig J: Teaching modules. *Nurs Management* (Dec) 1982; 13:38–40.

Fisher KM, MacWhinney B: AV autotutorial instruction: a review of evaluative research. *AV Comm Rev* 1976; 24:229–261.

Friesen L, Stotts NA: Retention of basic cardiac life support content: the effect of two teaching methods. *J Nurs Educ* 1984; 23:184–191.

Gentine M: Methods of teaching revisited: self-learning packages. *J Contin Educ Nurs* (May/June) 1980; 11:57–59.

Hinthorne R: Methods of teaching revisited: self-instructional modules. *J Contin Educ Nurs* (July/Aug) 1980; 11:37–39.

Keller FS: "Goodbye, teacher ... " *J Applied Behavior Analysis* 1968; 1:79–89.

Koniak D: Autotutorial and lecture-demonstration instruction: a comparative analysis of the effects upon students' learning of a developmental assessment skill. *West J Nurs Res* 1985; 7:80–100.

Kulik JA, Kulik CC, Cohen PA: A meta-analysis of outcome studies of Keller's personalized system of instruction. *Amer Psychologist* 1979; 34:307–318.

Layton J: Instructional packaging. *J Nurs Educ* (Nov) 1975; 14:26–30.

Linder S, Whitehurst C: Is there a novelty effect on student attitudes toward personalized instruction? *J Exper Educ* 1973; 42:42–44.

Mintzes JJ: The A-T approach 14 years later—a review of recent research. *J College Science Teaching* 1975; 4:247–252.

Mueller DJ: Evaluation of instructional materials and prediction of student success in a self-instructional section of an educational measurement course. *J Exper Educ* 1974; 42:53–55.

Myers LB, Greenwood SE: Use of traditional and autotutorial instruction in fundamentals of nursing courses. *J Nurs Educ* (March) 1978; 17:7–13.

Osborn WP, Thompson MA: Variables associated with student mastery of learning modules. *Communicating Nursing Research* 1976; 9:167–179.

Ostrow CL: The interaction of cognitive style, teaching methodology and cumulative GPA in baccalaureate nursing students. *J Nurs Educ* 1986; 25:148–155.

Pensivy BA: Traditional versus individualized nursing instruction. *J Nurs Educ* (Feb) 1977; 16:14–18.

Postlethwait SN, Novak J, Murray HT: *The Audio-Tutorial Approach to Learning,* 3d ed. Burgess, 1972.

Rufo KL: Effectiveness of self-instructional packages in staff development activities. *J Contin Educ Nurs* (May/June) 1985; 16:80–84.

Schiller WJ, Markle SM: Using the personalized system of instruction. Chapter 6 in: *On College Teaching*. Milton O & Associates (editors). Jossey-Bass, 1978.

Shavelson RJ, Munger MR: Individualized instruction: a systems approach. *J Educ Res* 1970; 63:263–268.

Stein RF et al: A multimedia independent approach. *Nurs Res* 1972; 21:436–447.

Thompson M: Learning: a comparison of traditional and autotutorial methods. *Nurs Res* 1972; 21:453–457.

Thompson MA: A systematic approach to module development. *J Nurs Educ* (Oct) 1978; 17:20–26.

Chapter 7

Learning Through Simulation

Simulation is, for most people, an enjoyable and stimulating way to learn. Because it is so enjoyable, it has been heralded by some as the best teaching method to come along since the lecture. There is no doubt about the usefulness of simulation; however, there are questions about whether it can live up to all of the claims that have been made about it. This chapter discusses three types of simulations that have been used in education—simulation exercises, simulation games, and role playing—and examines the value and role of each in the classroom.

For clarification, I should first define these three types of simulations:

Simulation exercise: A controlled representation of a piece of reality that learners can manipulate to better understand the corresponding real situation.

Simulation game: A game that represents real-life situations in which learners compete according to a set of rules in order to win or achieve an objective.

Role playing: A form a drama in which learners spontaneously act out roles in an interaction involving problems or challenges in human relations.

Simulation has been a teaching strategy for centuries. In the eighteenth century, German war games were developed for use in military academies. In the 1930s, role playing was experimented with, and in the 1940s the Link Trainer, a simulated aircraft cockpit, was used to teach pilots in the United States (Corbett & Beveridge, 1982). The first formal recognized use of simulation in education came in the 1960s when business, law, educational administration, and medicine all began to use various types of simulation formats.

Purpose of Simulation

Simulation is intended to help students practice decision-making and problem-solving skills and to develop human interaction abilities in a controlled and safe setting. By means of active involvement in a simulation exercise, a game, or a role-playing situation, the student achieves cognitive, affective, and psychomotor outcomes. Students have a chance to apply principles and theories they have learned and to see how and when these principles work. For example, a student may have read about the importance of eliciting an anxious patient's feelings and studied the techniques that can be used to do so. Role playing an interaction with an anxious patient (another student) can help the student see that these techniques work not only for authors of textbooks but for students, too. Another student may have learned about the nursing process from a series of lectures and audiovisuals, but the process only comes alive after the student applies it in a simulation case study drawn from the real world.

You may be thinking that this is all true, but the same outcomes can be achieved by means of clinical practice as well. Unarguably, the clinical area is the ultimate place to practice and apply the types of skills I am talking about, but the reality is that an instructor in the clinical laboratory often has ten students to help. He or she cannot be with each student through every interaction and problem-solving situation to guide and help with critical thinking skills. Also, not every student will encounter the "good" learning situations that teachers would like to provide each week.

In a classroom simulation, every student can experience the same patient situation and can be guided through the problem-solving process with all the expert help and peer support that he or she needs. Students can learn how to learn and can test various approaches in a setting where patients cannot be hurt and where wrong decisions can always be remedied. It is hoped that the learning gained from simulations in the classroom will transfer to the patient setting.

Uses of Simulation

Simulation techniques can be used to achieve many learning objectives. First, simulations can help nursing students gain skill in applying the nursing process. They can practice gathering and analyzing data, setting priorities, selecting and modifying interventions, and evaluating outcomes. They can learn to solve problems efficiently with minimal wasting of time and resources.

In the acquisition of communication skills, simulation techniques are almost unparalleled as an effective methodology. Students can put themselves in the shoes of others (patients, families, co-workers, supervisors, physicians) and learn something about these people's feelings and how to interact effectively with them. Students can gain acumen in problem areas of human relations. As they try out communication techniques, they get immediate feedback about how they affect other people.

Simulation is also an avenue for attitude change. Students who work through a simulation exercise or game or a role-playing situation may discover factors about certain people and situations that they never realized before and that will change their attitudes in the future. Constructive attitudes can lead to more productive and acceptable behavior.

Decision-making skills can be fostered via simulation. Students learn to make decisions by making decisions, not just by learning the theory of decision making. When they make decisions in a simulation of reality, they can see the immediate consequences. If the results are undesirable, they can backtrack and look at the factors that led them to a poor decision. The instructor and classmates (if a group is involved) can help the student gain insight into why a decision was effective or ineffective.

Simulation techniques can be applied to the learning of psychomotor skills. When students practice skills in a college laboratory using mannequins and hospital-type equipment, they are involved in a patient care simulation. (For further information about the value of this type of simulation, see Chapter 8.)

Finally, simulations can be used to evaluate student learning and competence. Written exams have been developed in a simulation format to test the application of knowledge. Such exams may also be used instead of or in addition to clinical performance exams. Further information on simulation examinations is provided later in this chapter.

Role of the Teacher

The teacher's role in simulations has three facets: planning, facilitating, and debriefing.

Planning begins with choosing or developing an appropriate simulation that will meet course objectives. Even if you can't find exactly what you want on the market, you may be able to adapt a commercially prepared simulation. Whether you purchase a simulation package or develop your own, you should try it out as much as possible before using it in class. If you are using a simulation game, ask other faculty to go through it with you. Case studies or other simulation exercises should be read carefully while you jot down notes about how you want to guide the students at various points or about questions you will want to ask during the simulation. Without a trial run, you may come up against some unanticipated snags in the classroom. Problems may be as basic as missing pieces from a board game or as complex as students having inadequate background knowledge to enable them to proceed through a simulation.

You will probably want to assign some reading for the students to do before class. Textbooks or library resources should be pointed out to students so that they can prepare for the simulation. If the theoretical background for the content has not been covered previously in class, students must be held responsible for coming to class prepared for the simulation. Written simulation exercises may be given to the students a few days before class so that they can familiarize themselves with the scenario and see what information they need beforehand.

Before class begins, you are responsible for preparing the environment. If a board game is to be played, tables and chairs should be set up. For discussion of simulation exercises, you may want to place chairs in a circle. Try not to waste class time in making environmental changes.

Some simulations will involve every member of the class; others will require only a few participants and many observers. All students should be involved in some way, as either actors, discussion members, players, scorekeepers, or observers. Totally uninvolved students soon become bored. Generally, students should be allowed to volunteer as participants. Forcing a reluctant student to take an active role does not usually serve any good purpose.

You should function as a facilitator during the actual progress of the simulation. After introducing the activity, you may take a backseat and talk relatively little. You may coach students who are trying to find their way through a sticky problem and encourage creative thinking and act as an information resource, but you should not be too quick to give advice or suggest solutions. Neither should you criticize thinking that doesn't coincide with your own. It is often a good idea to take notes during the class so that in later discussion you can refer back to specific strengths and weaknesses of the process, to interesting interpersonal exchanges, or to inconsistencies that no one else may have picked up.

The most important part of your role is the final discussion or debriefing session. If at all possible, the debriefing should occur immediately following the simulation when the information is fresh in everyone's mind. You should leave enough time to include several activities. First, you should briefly summarize what has taken place. Next, having the students explain what they did and why can be valuable. Self-analysis can help students gain insight into why they made certain decisions or took a specific course of action. A game player can explain his strategy, and a role player can analyze her enactment of a role. In simulations where emotions have run high, ventilation of feelings should be part of the debriefing. Finally, the observers should have an opportunity to give their impressions and perhaps to suggest what they would have done had they been the participants. As mentioned previously, feedback from the peer observers can engender lasting learning in the participants.

At the end of the discussion period you should point out how principles and concepts have been applied and how the experience ties in to the learning objectives. For example, a class may engage in a simulation exercise about a male patient who has cancer but who has not been told his diagnosis. His family knows but his friends do not. The situation unfolds with a series of interactions between patient and wife, patient and friends, physician and wife, nurses and physician, and nurse and patient. An objective of the simulation is understanding the interpersonal dynamics that occur when diagnoses are withheld from patients. You should help the class see how communication principles have been used and abused in the situation and how people react in varied ways when diagnoses are concealed.

This is a good place to bring in research related to the topic. In our example, research done on open and closed awareness contexts could be applied. This time can also be used to compare the simulation to the real world; when was it similar to and when did it depart from reality? You can point out which aspects of the simulation are applicable to future real situations and suggest adaptations that might be made to fit a variety of circumstances.

Types of Simulation Exercises

Simulation exercises include written simulations for individual and group use, audiovisual simulations, and the use of live simulated patients.

Written Simulations

Individual Uses   Written simulations for individual use are either paper-and-pencil or latent-image format. They are usually used to teach problem solving and decision making or to evaluate a student's ability to apply these skills. Written simulations for individual use can be developed for any level of student on any aspect of decision making. The format is quite flexible.

A paper-and-pencil simulation might be set up in a programmed learning style, where data about a patient or situation are given to the student and the student is asked to select from several options which course of action should be taken first or which problem is most evident in the opening data. The answers or responses to each of the items are on following pages. After receiving all the feedback on the first set of options, the student moves on to the next decision to be made.

The latent-image layout requires a special duplicating process, latent-image paper, and special markers. Introductory information is given, and the student is asked to make an initial decision about what to do, what data to collect, or which problem to work on first. However, the options to choose from and the responses or feedback from each option are on the same page. The responses are hidden from the student and are revealed only when the student rubs the marker over the indicated area to "uncover" the answer. A latent-image page might look like this:

Background Information

You are a nurse on the evening shift on a surgical unit in a general hospital. A young female patient was admitted earlier today with complaint of intermittent severe headaches. When you answer her light at 7 P.M., she states that her headache is more severe than it has ever been.

Select the option that you would carry out first:

1. Call the house physician   1. LATENT-IMAGE
    for an analgesic order.   RESPONSE

2. Take all vital signs.

3. Notify the attending
   physician.

4. Collect more information
   about the pain.

2. LATENT-IMAGE
   RESPONSE

3. LATENT-IMAGE
   RESPONSE

4. LATENT-IMAGE
   RESPONSE

Feedback is given on the uncovered response. If the wrong response is chosen, the student may be directed to uncover another response. Some questions may have several correct answers. In some cases, wrong selections that have irrevocable results may end the simulation for the learner.

Page and Saunders (1978) described the use of latent-image simulations in teaching the nursing process to first-year nursing students. They reported the development of two simulations, one dealing with the assessment phase, and the second covering both assessment and planning.

The Patient Management Problem (PMP) format is an example of a latent-image simulation that has been used in medical education and in nurse practitioner programs (Sherman et al, 1979). The PMP is a simulated encounter with a patient in a primary care setting in which the nurse must assess and try to alleviate patient problems. The nurse makes a series of inquiries and decisions and selects appropriate actions. Each selection impinges on subsequent selections in a realistic way.

The same simulation exercises used to *teach* clinical problem solving can be used to *evaluate* students' skill at problem solving. Students can take the simulations home and work on them the way they would work on any take-home or open-book test, or the simulations can be used for in-class examinations. Such examinations can be used to arrive at a portion of the clinical grade. They can also be used as a method of formative evaluation to assist students in identifying difficulties in decision making and problem solving.

Several researchers have investigated the reliability and validity of simulated clinical problem-solving examinations. Reliability of these simulations has not been a problem, but validity has. In 1968 deTornyay evaluated a clinical simulation that she used to evaluate students' problem-solving skills. She found "reasonable reliability" but tested only for content validity, which was present. Dincher and Stidger (1976) attempted to establish content, con-

struct, and concurrent validity of their written simulation designed
to evaluate clinical nursing judgment. They found little evidence
for construct and concurrent validity. The researchers concluded
that a test dealing with only one area of nursing knowledge cannot
be considered a valid measure of nursing judgment; a battery of
tests would be needed. McLaughlin, Carr, and Delucci (1981) reported evidence of content, concurrent, and construct validity of
two clinical simulation tests used to measure primary care management by nurses and physicians. In 1981, 1986, and 1988 Holzemer and colleagues attempted to establish validity of two different
PMPs. The first and last studies found only minimal support for the
validity of the PMP as a measure of problem solving. The 1986
report supplied information about the lack of evidence for criterion-related validity of another PMP. The authors conclude that
"because of the lack of criterion-related validity evidence reported
in the literature and by this study, educators should be cautious in
utilizing simulations for evaluation purposes" (1986; 289).

Group Uses   Written simulations can also be designed for group
use. When used for group discussion and problem solving, these
simulation exercises are often termed case studies. A case study
describes a patient situation, a health care situation, or a management or leadership situation that students are asked to analyze and
deal with using professional knowledge.

   One advantage to involving groups of students in case study
learning is that the students become used to the interaction among
(future) professionals. Few nurses work entirely independently.
Most work in institutions or group practices where their work
affects that of their colleagues and where groups of professional
people are working together to aid patients and clients.

   Case studies can range from the simple and short to the complex and lengthy. I devised a series of simple case studies for a
course I taught to freshmen associate degree nursing students that
covered basic human needs, common health problems, and related
nursing care. To teach students about the concepts of urinary control, urinary retention and incontinence, prevention of urinary infection, and urinary catheter care, I used the following case study:

Common Urinary Problems
Case Study

Mr. Richards, a 65-year-old retired man, is admitted
to your unit from the Emergency Department with a

medical diagnosis of urinary retention due to BPH (en-
larged prostate gland). A Foley catheter was inserted in
the ED to empty his bladder.

1. What would you assess on Mr. Richards?

2. What nursing care does he require?

Two days later Mr. Richards's Foley catheter is removed to see whether he can void, but after 6 hours he
still has not voided.

1. What assessments should you make now?

2. What nursing action could you take at this time?

3. What will determine how long you should wait be
    fore reinserting the catheter?

4. What nursing diagnoses would best describe Mr.
    Richards's problems at this time?

The following week Mr. Richards has surgery (prostat-
ectomy) and after two days his Foley catheter is again
removed. This time he keeps dribbling urine (lack of urinary control).

1. What assessments should you make at this time?

2. What nursing care is required now?

Placing this content about basic problems into real-life simulations helped the students see how such problems evolve and are
handled from a nursing perspective. It was the beginning of their
socialization process into the role of the nurse and initial use of the
nursing process.

The students were required to read a relevant chapter in their
textbook before coming to class and were told that we would apply
the information they read to a case study simulation. At the beginning of the semester we had made an agreement that when classes
such as this were scheduled, the students would be held accountable for coming to class prepared. If it became evident that many
students were not prepared, class would be dismissed and everyone would still be held responsible for the material. I only had to
dismiss a class once, because most students enjoyed the case studies and prepared for them.

At the other end of the spectrum are complex case studies that include interaction among many characters and manipulation of many variables. Daniel, Eigsti and McGuire developed a simulation of community caseload management that requires about 3 hours to complete. It describes a group of 25 families who have "maternal child health, communicable disease, mental health, health supervision, and direct nursing care needs" (1977; 28). Also included in the caseload are school assignments, agency audit committee work, responsibility for a well-child conference, an immunization clinic, and an inservice education program. The students are divided into groups of six and are assigned roles such as public health nurse, team leader, supervisor, licensed practical nurse, and home health aide. The student groups are asked to develop a monthly schedule to cover all of the work responsibilities in the total caseload. They have to consider frequency and intensity of home visits, priorities of care, educational preparation and roles of staff, and principles of delegation. When each group has completed its task, the entire class shares their plans and rationale for the care of the community.

Another complex simulation exercise is a simulated disaster called "Help," developed by Yantzie (1980). Learners in small groups act as triage teams to direct care during a disaster resulting from an explosion at a local cement factory. Participants decide which patients need priority care at the site, in what order they should be sent off in the ambulances, and what their disposition would be when they reach the hospital.

You can see that case studies can become very involved, but these types of simulations are invaluable because the same experiences may not be obtained in the limited clinical time available. This type of simulation may be valuable in inservice education as well.

Not all case studies that deal with complex situations take as much time as those just described. I have used some published vignettes of problems and conflicts experienced by nurse managers that involved management theory, communication principles, and change and conflict theories. The vignettes are very effective in helping students apply the conceptual material they have read and on which I have lectured, but each of these simulations takes only about 20 minutes to complete.

Features of Written Simulations   Written simulations, whether adapted to individual or group use, should include several features if they are to be effective. For one thing, they should generally be derived from real-life situations. Real cases are better because of the wealth of information from which to draw; fabricated simulations too often become just summaries of what supposedly happened. The more complex simulations, especially, should be based on real cases with all of the variables that were involved. Imagine how intrigued students are when they hear the actual outcome of the case compared to the outcomes that developed from their own manipulations.

Although you may already know the outcome of the real case, you should structure the exercise so that several different approaches to the solution could occur to the student. There should not be just one right answer; indeed, if that is the way your simulation develops, you probably made a poor selection of cases or provided too much information. By withholding some information near the end of the story, you can leave the solution open to several possibilities. The whole process is not unlike writing a mystery novel—give the reader enough clues to whet the appetite, but keep a few back so that he or she can speculate about what might happen.

The cases that you choose should not be esoteric or unique. Unique cases are tempting because they are the ones that tend to stick in one's memory. However, the purpose of simulations is rarely to teach about uncommon happenings; rather, it is to help students solve typical problems and confront commonplace data that they can transfer to their clinical practice. Save the unusual stories for times when you want to entertain or amaze your students.

Finally, it is important that the case be appropriate for the students' level of knowledge and experience. Cases that are too easy are boring, but those that are too difficult may defeat the objectives. Students should not have to spend hours in the library researching obscure information or data that they have never before encountered, nor should class time be wasted because students have no way of knowing the significance of certain data. Remember that the emphasis in simulations is on learning *process*; the learning of content should be a by-product.

Audiovisual Simulations

Incorporating audiovisuals into a simulation can add to its attractiveness and realism. Instead of the introductory information being written, it can be acted out or displayed and recorded on videotape or slides. In a nursing process simulation, the patient and the environment can be filmed, as can interactions between the patient and family or other professionals. Written questions and chart data can still be handed to the student to be used in conjunction with the media.

An entire simulation can be placed on videotape. Management vignettes can be dramatized and filmed. Questions can be posed for the viewers right on the screen, and the alternative outcomes, dependent on which approaches to a solution are chosen, can all be taped.

In computer simulations, which are covered in depth in Chapter 11, all patient or situation data can be given on the screen, where questions and answers can also appear. Graphics may be incorporated, which certainly add interest to the simulation.

Live Simulated Patients

Taking a patient history and doing a physical assessment for the first time is often a nerve-racking experience for learners. They are concerned about not forgetting things, about doing the right thing, and about trying to appear competent in front of the patient. Even though they may have practiced on classmates and family members ad nauseam, their first clinical encounter can be a real trial. Some schools have eased the transition from laboratory practice to real-world performance by the use of live simulated patients. These are people, sometimes nonnursing college students, who are paid to act as patients.

Lincoln, Layton and Holdman (1978) described their experience with simulated patients. The patients were healthy people, usually students, who were trained in the role they were to play. Each patient selected a role with which he or she would be comfortable, with the stipulation that it should not include problems that the person was actually experiencing, lest he or she fall into the role of real patient. Simulated patients used their own history as much as possible but memorized and added the elements of the history that had been created for the simulation.

The nursing students found the experience to be beneficial. They were still nervous at having to do the history and physical, especially because they were also being evaluated by an instructor, but believed that they would be much more relaxed and confident when meeting their first real patient.

McDowell et al (1984) worked with a similar program that was enthusiastically endorsed by faculty and students. They point out, however, that a simulation patient program requires extensive preparation time; in their case it was 50 hours of preparation the first time and somewhat less for subsequent classes. In addition, the cost of hiring the patients must be considered.

Simulation Games

Many educators are uncomfortable with the idea of using games in higher education. To some it may seem unprofessional, unconventional, and even unscholarly to have students "playing" in the classroom. Yet, for decades other educators have praised gaming as a productive and valuable asset in a teacher's collection of methods.

Some experts have advocated harnessing people's innate liking for and interest in games to educational purposes. Playing games is an integral part of childhood and adolescence, and there is no doubt that children learn a lot through their games. Shouldn't we in education exploit this natural way of learning, a way with which young people, especially, are familiar and comfortable?

Considering the proposition that people learn more when they are actively involved in the learning process, it would seem that games have potential as a vehicle of learning. But this vehicle differs in one important way from other teaching methods. In the process of game playing, the student's primary motivation is winning the game; learning the material becomes a secondary motivation (Hyman, 1974). Teachers have to understand and live with this fact if they use gaming strategies. It doesn't mean that students learn any less, just that they are learning in order to attain the goal of winning. However, students learn in order to achieve myriad other goals, too, so game playing can be looked on as a pragmatic way, among others, of motivating learners.

Games have been popular in education (though not in nursing education) since the 1960s. Wolf and Duffy (1979) explain why simulation games are not used more in nursing education. First, teachers were probably not exposed to this method when they were in nursing school or graduate school. It is always easier to use a method that one has personally experienced. Second, there are few commercially available simulation games in nursing, and those that exist are not well advertised. Third, it is usually impossible to "preview" simulation games; they must be purchased in order to try them out. Fourth, teachers may feel uneasy about justifying the use of games because it is difficult to evaluate the learning that takes place. Finally, it may be that many instructors find it difficult to devise games. Although many people could probably put together a simple word game, true simulation games that involve a game board or cards or physical action take a type of creative skill that few people possess.

Simulation games can be classified in various ways. It is helpful to know these classifications when looking for a game to meet certain objectives. One way of classifying games is to divide them into content games and process games (Ulione, 1983). *Content* games primarily provide cognitive factual information. They usually entail detailed roles and interactions and leave little room for improvisation. The rules are specified and held constant. *Process* games do contain factual information, but the emphasis is on affective learning and problem solving. The roles in the game are less prescribed and participants can improvise. The rules are not always explicit except to outline what is forbidden. These games involve complex group interactions.

Another taxonomy of games has been developed by Duke (1986). She classifies games into three categories: clinical, pathophysiologic, and psychosocial. *Clinical* process games are those that focus on nursing performance in a simulated clinical setting. *Pathophysiologic* process games provide content about pathophysiologic conditions. *Psychosocial* process games are those that primarily emphasize simulated psychosocial functioning. Duke classified all games that appeared in nursing journals between 1974 and 1984 according to her taxonomy (see Tables 7-1, 7-2, and 7-3).

In addition to the games listed in the tables, a few others have been published recently. "Blood Money" is a simulation game whose purpose is to increase students' sensitivity to clients' experiences within the health care system. Students play the roles of citizens who come into contact with the health care system and have problems with finances, quality of care, and inability to obtain necessary care (Joos, 1984).

The game "GUTS" is a card game similar to rummy that teaches factual information about digestion and the gastrointestinal system. The suits represent processes of digestion that are appropriate to various types of foods (French, 1980).

"The Response Is Right: A Communication Game Show" is an adaptation of "Communication Game" by Charron and Saxton (Eakes & Finnen, 1985). This simulation supplies clinical situations in which students are to select responses appropriate to a patient's

Table 7-1   Clinical Process Games and Simulations According to Structural Components

Source	Roles	Interactions	Rules	Goals	Criteria
Dearth and McKenzie, 1975 "Synoptics"	Prescribed: patient care committees, jury members	Team play—facilitator role-play; make decisions about problems	Both: fixed, changing, low ambiguity, emergent	Successfully play roles of various health professionals by making recommendations about problem clinical situation (receive approval from jury)	Time limit is approximately 1½ hours; team with fairest, most realistic recommendations wins; game ends when debriefing session completed
Daniel et al, 1977 "Caseload Management"	Prescribed: various community health nursing roles	Team play/role-play; make decisions about schedules; present plans	Both: fixed, changing, high ambiguity, emergent	Thoroughly develop one month schedule covering all responsibilities of a community health nurse	Time limit is approximately 3 hours; game ends when discussion complete about how schedules developed
Lincoln et al, 1978 and McDowell et al, 1978 "Simulated Patients"	Prescribed: nurse, patient	Peer play—evaluators/role-play; assess patient; synthesize findings	Prescriptive	Successfully perform physical assessment of simulated patient and formulate conclusions (accumulate score on rating scale)	Varying time limits for phases of simulation; game ends with completion of observed written performance behaviors

Table 7-1, continued   Clinical Process Games and Simulations According to Structural Components

Source	Roles	Interactions	Rules	Goals	Criteria
Woodbery and Hamric, 1981 "Mock Code" Carney, 1983 "Mock Ambu" Kaye et al, 1984 "Mega Code"	Prescribed: various members of code team	Team play—evaluator/role-play; make decisions about emergency problems	Prescriptive	Successfully play roles of various health team members while performing in a mock emergency situation	Game ends when team completes prescribed performance behaviors
Plasterer and Mills, 1983 "Management Game"	Prescribed: various members of an organization	Team play—facilitators/role-play; discuss decisions	Proscriptive	Successfully work within various organizational structure to experience behaviors contributing to organizational functioning	Playing time is approximately 1–1½ hours; game ends when debriefing session completed
Carney, 1983 "Ambu Race"	None prescribed	Team play—evaluator; locate and identify crash cart items	Prescriptive	Swiftly and correctly locate drugs and supplies on crash cart (acquire items in least amount of time)	Team that locates items in least amount of time wins

Table 7-1, continued   Clinical Process Games and Simulations According to Structural Components

Source	Roles	Interactions	Rules	Goals	Criteria
McClean, 1983 "Closing"	None prescribed	Team play— "Master of Ceremonies"/OR nurse; recognize breaks in sterile technique	Prescriptive	Swiftly and correctly identify breaks in sterile OR technique (accumulate assigned value points)	Team with greatest number of points wins
Smith, 1983 "Never a Dull Moment," "What a Morning"	Prescribed: staff midwives	Team play— facilitators/draw cards; role-play; make decisions about patient problems	Both: fixed, changing, low ambiguity, emergent	Accurately play roles of staff midwives by choosing appropriate nursing actions for selected wards of maternity patients	Total time limit is 40 minutes divided into two series of play; game ends when debriefing session completed
DeBella Baldigo, 1984 "Community Simulation Game"	Prescribed: program representatives, board of supervisors	Team play/role-play; present programs	Both: fixed, changing, low ambiguity, emergent	Accurately present the needs/requests of selected community groups to obtain city council approval	Time limit for presentation is 5 minutes; game ends when city council provides list of approved programs

Table 7-1, continued   Clinical Process Games and Simulations According to Structural Components

Source	Roles	Interactions	Rules	Goals	Criteria
Haggard, 1984 "The Disaster Game"	None prescribed	Peer play—judge/ draw cards; answer questions	Prescriptive	Correctly describe what should be done in various disaster situations (accumu- late points assigned by judge)	Player with greatest number of points wins
"Orientation Game"	None prescribed	Peer play— monitor/draw cards; progress on game board	Prescriptive	Correctly answer various hospital policy and procedure questions (progress on game board)	Playing time is approximately 1 hour; first player to reach "payroll office" wins

* Prescriptive = Fixed role behaviors, constant interactions, low ambiguity in role delineation, specified patterns.
   Proscriptive = Flexible role behaviors, changing interactions, high ambiguity in role delineation, emergent patterns.

Source: Adapted from Duke ES: A taxonomy of games and simulations for nursing education. *J Nurs Educ* 1986; 25:197–206.

Table 7-2 Pathophysiologic Process Games and Simulations According to Structural Components

Source	Roles	Interactions	Rules	Goals	Criteria
Crancer and Maury-Hess, 1980 "It's a G.A.S."	None prescribed	Peer play/draw cards; answer questions	Prescriptive	Correctly answer discussion questions about general adaption syndrome (accumulate assigned value points)	No time limit; player with greatest number of points wins
"The Pluses and Minuses of Life"	None prescribed	Peer play/draw cards; answer questions	Prescriptive	Correctly answer multiple-choice questions about fluid and electrolyte, acid-base balance (accumulate assigned value points)	No time limit; player with greatest number of points wins
"How Sweet It Isn't"	None prescribed	Team play/draw cards; relay facts: score opposite team	Both: fixed, constant, low ambiguity, emergent	Correctly supply data about diabetic content (accumulate points assigned by opposite team)	Time limit for each answer is 3 minutes; team with most points wins
"Positive Pressure"	None prescribed	Peer play/draw cards; group cards	Prescriptive	Correctly match concepts to form sets of respiratory disease, pathophysiologic symptoms, and treatment	No time limit; game ends when all cards are grouped into sets of four

Table 7-2, continued Pathophysiologic Process Games and Simulations According to Structural Components

Source	Roles	Interactions	Rules	Goals	Criteria
"K.I.S.S."	None prescribed	Peer play/throw dice; answer questions; progress on game board	Prescriptive	Correctly answer questions about cardiovascular problems/blood dyscrasias (progress on game board)	No time limit; first player to advance out of "heart" to end of one "extremity" wins
"Vertigo"	None prescribed	Team play—score-keeper/draw cards; answer questions	Prescriptive	Correctly answer questions about neurologic dysfunctions (accumulate assigned value points)	No time limit; team with greatest number of points wins
Kolb, 1983 "3-North"	None prescribed	Peer or team play—card dealer/draw cards; synthesize data; plan care; score opposite team	Both: fixed, constant, low ambiguity, emergent	Successfully complete nursing process using fluid/electrolyte problems in pediatric patients (accumulate assigned value points from cards/opposing team)	Time limit for each phase of play is 15–20 minutes; player or team with most points wins

Table 7-2, continued Pathophysiologic Process Games and Simulations According to Structural Components

Source	Roles	Interactions	Rules	Goals	Criteria
Marcus, 1983 "Navigating the Inner Sea"	None prescribed	Peer play—moderator/ throw dice; draw cards; answer questions; "build kidney"	Prescriptive	Correctly answer question or discuss chance answers about renal pathophysiology (acquire kidney components)	Playing time is approximately 50 minutes; first player to build complete kidney wins

* Prescriptive = Fixed role behaviors, constant interactions, low ambiguity in role delineation, specified patterns.
Proscriptive = Flexible role behaviors, changing interactions, high ambiguity in role delineation, emergent patterns.

Source: Adapted from Duke ES: A taxonomy of games and simulations for nursing education. *J Nurs Educ* 1986; 25:197–206.

Table 7-3   Psychosocial Process Games According to Structural Components

Source	Roles	Interactions	Rules	Goals	Criteria
Chaisson, 1977 "Life Cycle"	Prescribed: senior citizens, significant others	Team play—managers/throw dice; role-play; progress on game board	Both: fixed, changing, low ambiguity, emergent	Authentically play roles of older persons or their significant others in real-life situations (progress on game board)	Playing time is approximately 10 hours divided into 3 sessions; game ends when debriefing session completed
Clark, 1977 "Psychiatric Nurse-Patient Relationship Game"	Prescribed: nurse-student, patient-teacher	Peer play/draw cards; respond to simulations; score answers	Prescriptive	Therapeutically respond in simulated psychiatric nurse–patient situations (accumulate assigned value points with chances to recover missed points)	Game ends when posttest completed
Farley and Fay, 1983 and Bonstelle and Govoni, 1984 "Into Aging"	Prescribed: elderly person	Peer play—four facilitators/draw cards; role-play, progress through "lifestyles"	Both: flexible, constant, low ambiguity, emergent	Representatively play role as an older person (progress through independent, semidependent, dependent lifestyles)	Playing time is approximately 1–2 hours; game ends when debriefing session completed

Table 7-3, continued   Psychosocial Process Games According to Structural Components

Source	Roles	Interactions	Rules	Goals	Criteria
Engelke, 1983 "T.E.A.C.H."	Prescribed: nurses, patients with neuro deficits, ancillary staff	Team play—faculty judge/plan education; role-play; draw figures	Both: fixed, changing, low ambiguity, emergent	Successfully play role of "nurse educator" so that "handicapped patient" can be taught to draw an unseen geometric figure	Playing time is approximately 40 minutes; team with most accurate set of geometric drawings wins
Dowd, 1983 "Blind Simulation"	Prescribed: sighted person, unsighted person	Peer play/role-play; watch videotape of experiences	Both: fixed, changing, low ambiguity, emergent	Accurately play role of someone who is blind to experience his/her disability	Playing time is approximately 2½ hours; game ends when debriefing session completed
Astill-McNish, 1984 "Where Do We Get Our Attitudes About Aging?"	None prescribed	Peer play—moderator/recall events; discuss feelings	Proscriptive	Accurately recall positive/negative experiences with elderly to recognize effects on personal attitudes	Time limit is 1 hour; game ends when group completes discussion about how experiences affect attitudes toward elderly
"Aging . . Moi?"	Prescribed: yourself at 72 years old	Peer play—moderator/imagine about aging; draw self; discuss feelings	Proscriptive	Accurately relate aging process to own lifestyle by drawing picture of self at 72 years old	Time limit is 1½ hours; game ends when group completes discussion about feelings from exercise

Table 7-3, continued   Psychosocial Process Games According to Structural Components

Source	Roles	Interactions	Rules	Goals	Criteria
"Losses and What They Do"	None prescribed	Peer play—moderator/list people, possessions; eliminate items on list; discuss feelings	Proscriptive	Accurately recognize how a series of losses influence self-esteem	Time limit is 1 hour; game ends when group finishes relating exercise to experiences of many elderly
"Who Am I Anyway"	None prescribed	Peer play—moderator/recall event; discuss feelings	Proscriptive	Accurately convey an anecdote from one's past that reveals other aspects about self	Time limit is 1½ hours; game ends when group finishes relating exercise to caring for those in sick role
"Come to Tea in the Day Room"	Prescribed; elderly person, caregivers	Peer play—moderator/role-play; discuss feelings	Both: fixed, changing, low ambiguity, emergent	Accurately play role of elderly person or his/her caregiver in an institutional setting	Playing time is approximately 2 hours; game ends when debriefing session completed

* Prescriptive = Fixed role behaviors, constant interactions, low ambiguity in role delineation, specified patterns.
Proscriptive = Flexible role behaviors, changing interactions, high ambiguity in role delineation, emergent patterns.

Source: Adapted from Duke ES: A taxonomy of games and simulations for nursing education. *J Nurs Educ* 1986; 25:197–206.

feelings. The original game is a board game for two to six players, but it was revised to the game show format for a class of 165 students.

Clark (1986) developed a health planning game in which community leaders, including nurses, meet to discuss health care problems in the community and decide how available resources will be spent on these problems. Directions for this simulation game are included in the journal article.

This list of games is by no means exhaustive. A number of books contain compilations of games, some of which are health related and many of which could be adapted to nursing (Joos, 1984). These books include *Guide to Simulations/Games for Education and Training* by Horn and Cleaves (1980).

Role Playing

Recall from the beginning of this chapter that role playing is a form of drama in which learners spontaneously act out roles in an interaction involving problems or challenges in human relations. The word *spontaneously* is important to understand in this activity. The participants do not have any scripts to follow, nor do they rehearse. They are given a written or verbal explanation of the simulated situation and are expected to have enough general knowledge about the situation to understand the roles to which they have been assigned.

This teaching method is effective in helping nursing students gain skill in interpersonal and therapeutic relationships and in teaching them how to handle interpersonal conflicts. It enables them to step into the shoes of others and therefore gain some insight into the perspectives of other people. Role playing may be a means of helping people develop the quality of empathy. It can assist them in understanding social problems of groups of people who are different from themselves. Many teachers have also used role playing to allow students to prepare for upcoming real situations, such as job interviews, evaluation interviews, patient counseling sessions, and so on.

A teacher can plan for role playing and prepare some instructions that will be given to the participants, or the teacher can use this strategy on the spur of the moment when a question arises about peoples' reactions, responses, or feelings related to whatever topic is being discussed in class that day.

Most role-playing scenarios last only about 3 to 5 minutes; it doesn't take long to illustrate one particular aspect of human inter-action. The instructor may choose to take more time, though, and have several sets of participants act out the same roles or have them switch roles after a few minutes. Those students who are not participating should be observing for nonverbal behavior, response patterns, examples of implementation of principles, and so on.

When the time for discussion arrives, talk should be steered away from self-criticism or peer criticism of the acting and instead focused on the enactment of the roles. The students should be critiquing the characters that are dramatized, not the people who are doing the acting.

Role playing has long been used to teach therapeutic communi-cation skills. An introduction to such a simulation usually begins something like this:

Background Information

Ms. Holden is a 62-year-old who has been hospital-ized for a week with gastrointestinal bleeding. Surgery is being considered, but Ms. Holden is reluctant to have surgery because she is concerned about who will care for her 87-year-old mother, who is at home. Ms. Holden says to you, her nurse, "I just can't seem to make a decision about this operation."

One student would enact the role of Ms. Holden, another would take the part of the nurse, and the interaction would proceed. Videotaping the session can be helpful for reference use during the discussion period.

"Land of Suria," a role-playing simulation by Dahl (1984), is a fairly well structured simulation designed to give students experi-ence in communicating with people from a culture not previously known to them. Two groups of students take part: one group play the Surians, who are concerned about a health problem resulting from urban renewal; the other group are health care workers who have never before met the Surians but who will try to discover what their problems are. This is a good example of a role-playing situation for the purpose of learning appreciation of cultural roles and transcultural interaction.

Reichman and Weaver-Meyers (1984) describe a simulation they wrote called "Glaucoma and Cataracts: A Nurse-Patient Simulation." In this program, one student plays the role of an almost blind patient and another plays her nurse. Both players are given considerable background information, and the patient is supplied with a pair of clouded swimmer's goggles. The pair are instructed to carry out certain activities while they are in their roles. At the end of the simulation, the students reverse roles.

It is relatively easy for a teacher to devise role-playing simulations that will help him or her meet many different class objectives. It is important, though, to keep those objectives in mind. If the instructor wants learners to gain practice in handling conflict situations between nurses and other health care professionals, for example, he or she should write a situation in which an interpersonal conflict is evident and in which the learners will be able to use the principles of conflict resolution in their role enactment.

Advantages of Simulations

Educators who have used simulations claim many advantages to this method. Some of these claims are backed by research, some are not, but the accumulated evidence of the experience of many educators does give weight to their assumptions.

Reid (1976) believes that an advantage to simulation is that it reduces the complexities of real-life situations to a level that can be dealt with by beginners. Subjecting a novice in nursing to a patient situation with multiple interacting variables and asking that student to enact the professional role is ludicrous. By controlling some of the variables, the situation is still close to reality but is slightly simplified. The student is not overwhelmed and can concentrate on reacting to a few variables at a time.

An advantage of simulation emphasized by many educators is its motivating properties. Because simulation techniques are fun and interesting, they can motivate people to learn. Students see how theories that sometimes seem dry and sterile can really be useful and absorbing. Simulation appeals to both slow and fast learners and apparently is effective for all types of students.

Peer learning, known to be an effective way to learn, plays a role in most simulation techniques. Students often discuss simulation exercises in a group or act out parts of the situation while others are observing. Watching others succeed or fail can help the observers see which strategies work and why, and the observers help the participants by commenting on their performance. Everyone can learn from the people who are successful in solving simulated problems or from players who win a game. Students also learn from the faculty member who is guiding the simulation and leading discussions, but it is possible that students learn more from their peers than from the instructor.

Simulations allow students to make mistakes in decision making and problem solving and in interpersonal relationships—mistakes that might be catastrophic in the workplace. They make these mistakes with impunity except for possible blows to the ego. It would be nice if simulations could be structured so that all possible mistakes would be made and students would never make those same mistakes in the real world. But by making at least some mistakes, students learn about types of pitfalls and how to avoid them. They also learn ways of extricating themselves from ticklish situations.

Dekkers and Donatti (1981) mention that simulation enables the student to acquire concrete meanings for abstract terms. Teachers talk of concepts such as "discharge planning," "interdisciplinary collaboration," and "therapeutic use of self," but these concepts remain abstract until they are applied in a simulation. The student suddenly sees that discharge planning means something as concrete as helping Mrs. Smith figure out where to buy surgical supplies in her neighborhood, or that setting a goal to encourage a patient to express his feelings is one thing but saying the right things and in the right way so that the patient will actually be encouraged to speak is another. Students need this application of concepts and abstract theories. If the simulations are realistic enough, the student should be able to transfer the learning to real clinical settings.

The last important advantage to this teaching method is that it encourages creative and divergent thinking. Students can experiment with a whole gamut of solutions to a problem or with a variety of nursing interventions to meet a patient's need. They can test some outside possibilities that would not be feasible in the real world. Instead of just wondering "What if . . . " they can carry each alternative to its logical conclusion to see what the outcomes might be. When a group of students are all working on the same simulation and many ideas are being contributed, they are often amazed at how many ways a single situation can be approached.

Disadvantages of Simulation

Simulation methodology also has its limitations and drawbacks, although none of them presents insurmountable obstacles to the method's effective use. One frequently cited disadvantage is that simulation is costly in terms of both time and money. The few published simulations or games applicable to nursing can cost hundreds of dollars each. An educator who wants to devise a simulation or game can spend weeks or months in doing so. That isn't to say, of course, that very simple simulations cannot be devised in a fraction of that time.

Simulation techniques also consume a lot of classroom time. Hours can be spent in working through a case study or playing a game. Some teachers are reluctant to spend so much time on simulations because the students are usually not learning a lot of content in those hours; they are essentially learning *process*. Teachers often assume that a certain amount of factual content must be covered in a course, even at the expense of application of that content. If they insist on lecturing on all of the required content, no time may be left over for strategies like simulation.

On the other hand, simulation techniques can be overused. Too much simulation in a nursing course would preclude the acquisition of necessary factual content and would result in boredom, as would be the case with overuse of any method. If simulation is to retain its motivational advantage, it should be used sparingly.

Any instructor who engages a class in simulation activities can expect occasional high noise levels and increased activity in the classroom. As the class becomes involved in the simulation and feelings are activated, voices will be raised, laughter may ensue, and several conversations may be going on at a time. If the physical facilities warrant quietness in the classroom, the teacher may have to limit or adapt the use of simulations.

Simulation strategies are most effective when good group dynamics exist in a class. If the students who are working on a simulation exercise, game, or role playing do not get along well or are not comfortable with each other, the entire process may be hampered. An instructor should assess the group dynamics in a classroom before introducing some of these techniques. It may be wise not to initiate simulations too early in the semester; the students should be given time to become comfortable as a group. Remember that taking part in simulations can be a risky business for students. They are being asked to apply their knowledge and interpersonal skills in front of their peers. They open themselves up to possible criticism, and some are afraid they will make fools of themselves. If the members of the group do not trust each other, their risk taking will be minimal.

It is possible that emotions may be aroused to an undesirable degree, especially with role playing. A student may identify with a particular role, or the simulation may evoke painful memories. The teacher should watch carefully and be aware if students are getting carried away.

Simulation games also have some unique disadvantages built into them. As Walljasper points out, learning sometimes takes a backseat if the level of competition becomes too high and "participants start comparing scores, not ideas, or devote more energy to arguing about rules and infractions than to addressing the subject . . . " (1982; 16). Some players may focus so much on winning that all else is sacrificed, and for some the fear of losing suspends the ability to learn. Teachers must constantly focus on the learning outcomes and sometimes downplay the competition.

Not every instructor feels comfortable using simulation strategies. Because the class can be rather unstructured, the teacher must be flexible and able to change gears quickly to suit the needs of the situation. Simulation exercises, especially, can take off in unsuspected directions, and the instructor has not only to follow but sometimes to lead the students down these new paths.

If you choose to use this teaching method, you won't always have all the information you need in front of you on a notepad. You will have to draw on your knowledge and experience to answer questions the students may raise. You have to be prepared to defend your answers and suggestions. Students may challenge your solutions and demand to know why your approach is any better than theirs. The more secure you are in working with the students in a democratic manner, the better off you will be with simulation techniques.

Finally, the processes and outcomes of simulation methods are not always predictable. Unless the objectives are clear to all involved and unless the instructor builds in some controls to keep the students on the right path, the exercise may veer off into tangents, and objectives will not be met. The teacher sometimes walks a tightrope, trying on the one hand to allow the participants to work through a simulation with a lot of freedom so that discovery learning and independent problem solving are taking place, and on the other hand attempting to maintain some influence on the process and keep the group to the task at hand. Even if the teacher does his or her best, there is no certainty that all hoped for outcomes will be achieved.

Research on Simulation

Research has been conducted on all three aspects of simulation discussed in this chapter: simulation exercises, simulation games, and role playing. The dependent variables that have been investigated include student response to simulations, cognitive and affective learning, and student motivation.

Most research has revealed a positive student response to learning by simulation. Cherryholmes (1966) summarized the results of six early studies of simulation by saying that students evidenced a higher degree of interest in simulations than in conventional teaching methods. Many authors of simulation games have surveyed student opinions after the games were played and found positive reactions (French, 1980; Hamm & Brodt, 1982). When Norris tested student reactions to being taught communication skills by means of lecture or by role playing, she found that the role-playing group, more than the lecture group, said that "the method promoted active involvement, held their interest and was a preferred learning approach" (1984; 104).

Other studies have focused on the issue of whether cognitive learning is achieved through the simulation method. In the six studies reviewed by Cherryholmes (1966), there was no support for the belief that students being taught via simulation learned any more or less than those being taught by conventional methods. A study conducted by Stuck and Manatt (1970) in which one group of student teachers was taught school law by means of simulation and another group by means of lecture revealed that the simulation group scored significantly higher on a posttest. Wentworth and Lewis summarized research done in the late 1960s and early 1970s on simulation gaming and concluded, "if content learning is the major instructional goal, then it appears that other activities and techniques . . . may be equally or even more effective" (1973; 438).

Greenblat writes that it is difficult to identify what type of learning takes place with simulation. She says, "many researchers report that learning is in general terms. They suggest that students gain in awareness . . . but find it difficult to specify just what the content of the learning is" (1973; 73). When Dekkers and Donatti

(1981) performed a meta-analysis of 93 studies, they found no evidence that simulation activities result in greater cognitive gains than other teaching strategies.

Considerable research evidence does support the contention that simulation methods result in affective learning, especially attitude change. Fisher (1978) discovered that attitude change was greater among college administrators who participated in a simulation than among those who participated in a seminar with the same content. Greenblat (1973) summarized several studies revealing that more liberal and more empathetic attitudes developed as a result of simulation exercises and role playing. Dekkers and Donatti's meta-analysis suggests that positive attitude change results more from the use of simulations than from lectures.

The claim that simulations motivate learners has been substantiated in several studies. Seidner's summary of recent simulation research states that several researchers have found simulations to be "particularly effective in motivating students who normally were uninterested in school, or who tended not to work up to their capabilities" (1976; 236). Most of the testimonials about the motivating properties of simulations are from anecdotal evidence— reports of teachers who used simulations and who claim that students became very interested and involved and even wanted to extend the class sessions (Greenblat, 1973).

An interesting approach to simulation research was taken by Manderino et al (1986). They developed a simulation of a cardiac arrest situation and tested it to see whether students would react in the simulation as they would in real life. The criteria they used were measurements of state anxiety and physiologic anxiety. The participants indeed experienced significant manifestations of stress even though they realized they were only involved in a simulation, giving support to the validity of the simulation. Further validity testing of nursing simulations, whether used for teaching or evaluation purposes, is needed so that teachers can be confident that the activities do simulate reality.

Simulation research has suffered from many methodological problems, including problems in research design such as giving only posttests and having no control group. Samples have often been unrepresentative, and generalizations drawn from the studies have been too broad. Yet these studies have value if they are read with a critical eye. What is needed, as is the case with research into other teaching strategies, is not just more studies comparing this method with others but studies related to how simulations can best be structured and applied. In which situations and for which students do they function best? Are simulations indeed able to teach process variables? Many questions still need to be investigated.

In the future we will see a continued burgeoning of simulation use in nursing education. Research must keep up with application of this method to give it further scientific foundation.

References

Cherryholmes CH: Some current research on effectiveness of educational simulations: implications for alternative strategies. *American Behavioral Scientist* 1966; 10:4–7.

Clark HM: A health planning simulation game. *Nurse Educator* (July/Aug) 1986; 11:16–19.

Corbett NA, Beveridge P: Simulation as a tool for learning. *Top Clin Nurs* (Oct) 1982; 4:58–67.

Dahl J: Structured experience: a risk-free approach to reality-based learning. *J Nurs Educ* 1984; 23:34–37.

Daniel L, Eigsti DG, McGuire SL: Teaching caseload management. *Nurs Outlook* 1977; 25:27–29.

Dekkers J, Donatti S: The integration of research studies on the use of simulation as an instructional strategy. *J Educ Res* 1981; 74:424–427.

deTornyay R: Measuring problem-solving skills by means of the simulated clinical nursing problem test. *J Nurs Educ* (Aug) 1968; 7:3–8, 34–35.

Dincher JR, Stidger SL: Evaluation of a written simulation format for clinical nursing judgment. *Nurs Res* 1976; 25:280–285.

Duke ES: A taxonomy of games and simulations for nursing education. *J Nurs Educ* 1986; 25:197–206.

Eakes GG, Finnen R: Modification of a simulation game for use in a large group setting. *J Nurs Educ* 1985; 24:170–171.

Fisher CF: Being there vicariously by case studies. Pages 258–285 in: *On College Teaching*. Jossey-Bass, 1978.

French P: Academic gaming in nurse education. *J Adv Nurs* 1980; 5:601–613.

Greenblat CS: Teaching with simulation games. *Teaching Sociology* 1973; 1:62–83.

Hamm BH, Brodt D: GUTS: Teaching assertiveness skills by simulation and gaming. *Nurs Res* 1982; 31:246–247.

Holzemer WL, McLaughlin FE: Concurrent validity of clinical simulations. *West J Nurs Res* 1988; 10:73–83.

Holzemer WL et al: Simulations as a measure of nurse practitioners' problem-solving skills. *Nurs Res* 1981; 30:139–144.

Holzemer WL, Resnick B, Slichter M: Criterion-related validity of a clinical simulation. *J Nurs Educ* 1986; 25:286–290.

Horn RE, Cleaves A (editors): *The Guide to Simulations/Games for Education and Training*, 4th ed. Sage, 1980.

Hyman RT: *Ways of Teaching*, 2d ed. Lippincott, 1974.

Joos IR: A teacher's guide for using games and simulations. *Nurse Educator* (Autumn) 1984; 9:25–29.

Lincoln R, Layton J, Holdman H: Using simulated patients to teach assessment. *Nurs Outlook* 1978; 26:316–320.

Manderino MA et al: Evaluation of a cardiac arrest simulation. *J Nurs Educ* 1986; 25:107–111.

McDowell J et al: Evaluating clinical performance using simulated patients. *J Nurs Educ* 1984; 23:37–39.

McLaughlin FE, Carr JW, Delucci KL: Measurement properties of clinical simulation tests. *Nurs Res* 1981; 30:5–9.

Norris J: Teaching communication skills: Effects of two methods of instruction and selected learner characteristics. *J Nurs Educ* 1986; 25:102–106.

Page GG, Saunders S: Written simulation in nursing. *J Nurs Educ* (April) 1978; 17:28–32.

Reichman SL, Weaver-Meyers P: Glaucoma and cataracts: a nurse-patient simulation for nursing students. *J Nurs Educ* 1984; 23:314–315.

Reid N: Simulations, games and case studies. *Education in Chemistry* 1976; 12:82–83.

Seidner CJ: Teaching with simulations and games. Pages 217–250 in: *The Psychology of Teaching Methods*. Gage NL (editor). University of Chicago Press, 1976.

Sherman JE et al: A simulated patient encounter for the family nurse practitioner. *J Nurs Educ* (May) 1979; 18:5–15.

Stuck DL, Manatt RP: A comparison of audio-tutorial and lecture methods of teaching. *J Educ Res* 1970; 63:414–418.

Ulione MS: Simulation gaming in nursing education. *J Nurs Educ* 1983; 22:349–351.

Walljasper D: Games with goals. *Nurse Educator* 1982; 7:15–18.

Wentworth DR, Lewis DR: A review of research on instructional games and simulations in social studies education. *Social Education* 1973; 37:432–440.

Wolf MS, Duffy, ME: *Simulations/Games: A Teaching Strategy for Nursing Education*. NLN Publication #23-1756, 1979.

Yantzie N: HELP! Simulated disaster game. *Canadian Nurse* (June) 1980; 76:33–36.

Chapter 8

Teaching Psychomotor Skills

The amount of emphasis placed on the teaching of psychomotor skills has waxed and waned over the past few decades. Pressured by the increase in technology and nursing science, faculty have felt compelled to cut some things out of the curriculum in order to add new information. One of the more expendable areas of content has been clinical psychomotor skills.

The 1980s saw a resurgence of interest in teaching clinical skills in basic curricula. Inservice educators have long expressed the belief that new graduates should have more skill competence than they usually do. The patient's right to safe nursing care provided by skilled practitioners is being talked about more than ever, and students themselves are becoming increasingly vocal about their need to graduate with more than a modicum of psychomotor skills. Students and new graduates, regardless of the breadth and depth of their knowledge, feel insecure and incompetent unless their technical skills are fairly well developed.

However, in an age when clinical sites are in some places being reduced and clinical time is at a premium, faculty are often hard pressed to teach additional skills or to provide more practice, and they are searching for more efficient and effective ways of teaching psychomotor skills.

In the past, students learned how to perform a great number of skills in the nursing arts lab of the school of nursing. The instructor demonstrated the skill, and learners were given considerable practice time and were then required to give a return demonstration. Soon thereafter, the learner had an opportunity to apply most of the skills in the hospital. There is no doubt that the majority of learners reached skill mastery rather quickly by these methods.

But today, teachers must find alternative ways to teach technical skills because they don't usually have the luxuries of a lot of lab time, clinical time, and all the practice space and equipment that previously existed. So they must review their knowledge about how people learn psychomotor skills and apply it in new ways.

Phases of Skill Learning

The literature describes several models of how people learn to perform psychomotor skills. The model proposed by Gentile (1972) is logical and easy to understand. Gentile divides skill learning into two main stages: "getting the idea of the movement" and "fixation/diversification." Within these two main phases are several cognitive and behavioral patterns.

Stage One: Getting the Idea of the Movement

The initial step in getting the idea of the movement is having a goal. That is, the learner is confronted with a clear-cut need or problem. For example, the need may be to catheterize a patient's bladder and the goal is to learn to do so.

Many stimuli affect the learner and his or her environment at this point, some of which relate to the goal and some not. All stimuli that affect goal accomplishment are called *regulatory stimuli* and must be attended to. The learner must devote *selective attention* to the regulatory stimuli in order to form an effective plan of movements that will attain the goal. Learners often have difficulty in determining which stimuli are relevant and which are not. In the case of learning urinary catheterization, the student must selectively attend to the necessary equipment; the verbal, visual, or written instructions; the position of the patient; the anatomy of the area; the need for privacy; and so on. Stimuli that must be tuned out are irrelevant talk and noise in the environment, unnecessary equipment, and stimuli from the patient and from the nurse's own body, such as an itchy nose.

If the skill to be learned is a closed skill, the learner's task in sorting out stimuli is not too difficult. A *closed skill* is one in which environmental conditions and relevant stimuli remain stable throughout and possibly across performances. An example of a closed skill is handwashing or making an unoccupied bed. On the other hand, an *open skill* takes place in a changing environment, and the regulatory stimuli vary throughout the performance of the skill. A catheterization is an open skill because the patient may continue to talk, cry, or move during the procedure. Giving an injection to a squirming infant is another prime example of an open skill. Open skills, then, are more difficult for the learner because of unpredictable and changing stimuli to which attention must be given.

Once the learner recognizes and attends to the necessary stimuli, he or she will begin to plan movements to meet the environmental demands. Such a *motor plan* is a general mental preconception of what movements will be required to attain the goal. The learner then executes this motor plan with greater or lesser success.

After the skill (or a subset of the skill) is performed, the learner receives feedback regarding its execution. The feedback may be intrinsic ("I knew as soon as I started to touch the sheet that I was making a mistake") or extrinsic (the patient became upset, no urine came through the catheter, the instructor frowned). As a result of the feedback, the learner makes a decision about whether the goal was met and what to do next.

Stage Two: Fixation/Diversification

If the goal was not met, the learner needs to again go through the process of getting the idea of the movement. When the performance is successful, however, the learner proceeds to the stage of fixation/diversification. During this time, the learner refines his or her performance, alters it as necessary, and in the process fixes it in memory. This stage includes varying amounts of practice that will help the learner achieve the desired level of skill.

Role of the Teacher in Skill Learning

The teacher's role begins in the first stage, when the learner is confronted by a problem and consequently develops a goal. The teacher ensures that the goal and the intended outcomes are clear in the learner's mind. If urinary catheterization is the skill to be learned, the instructor teaches the nature of the skill, the need for accurate insertion under sterile conditions, and the outcome of bladder emptying.

Along with clearly establishing the goal, the teacher may have to ensure an adequate motivational level in the learner. This is usually not a problem with nursing students; they are eager to learn skills like catheterization. But sometimes learners do not have sufficient motivation to sustain them to the point of skill mastery. I have seen this happen with such less "exciting" skills as range of motion exercises, specimen collection, and patient positioning. Learners don't find these skills very interesting and may not see them as important, which means that the teacher must help them see the value and usefulness of these procedures.

The next task for the educator is to help the learner recognize and attend to the regulatory stimuli. Assisting the learner to recognize and attend to relevant stimuli can be done in several ways. The teacher can provide a verbal or written outline of the steps of the procedure and their rationale, or can present a live or taped demonstration. The instructor can use guided discovery and problem solving at certain points to help the learner reason out the next step in the procedure. Whatever the method, the learner must become familiar with the steps of a procedure, the equipment to be used, and the impact of the environment on skill performance.

Controlling the Learning Environment

The instructor must make decisions about how the learning and practice environments should be structured. One approach is to simplify the environment as much as possible by reducing or eliminating nonregulatory stimuli and holding regulatory stimuli constant. This approach would tend to make all skills fit the closed-skill mode. Using urinary catheterization as the example again, the instructor might teach the skill using a mannequin in the college laboratory, with a minimum number of people around, curtains pulled around the bed, and no distracting noise. The disadvantage of simplifying the environment in this way is that when the learner eventually has to perform the skill in the real clinical world with multiple changing stimuli, he or she may be at a disadvantage. The learner may have difficulty transferring what was learned in the closed mode to the open mode found in a clinical site.

The opposite approach is to teach skills, especially open skills, in as realistic a setting as possible. The student might learn the cognitive aspects of the procedure in the classroom or through independent study; however, demonstration and performance would be done in a clinical setting. With this method, the learner would perform the skill for the first time on an actual patient needing a catheterization and would be forced to cope with all of the changing stimuli that usually attend such occasions. The drawbacks to this procedure are obvious. The patient is subjected to treatment by a person who is an absolute novice in the skill, even though supervised, and this fact may become evident to the patient. Also, the student would probably be trying to cope with considerable anxiety while trying to learn the skill. Finally, a lengthy time lag may occur between learning the cognitive aspects of the skill and actually putting it into practice in the clinical area, which is detrimental to learning.

A middle road between these two approaches is difficult but not impossible to achieve. It is possible to teach skills in a college lab but also to discuss the kinds of environmental changes learners can expect when in the clinical area. The teacher can demonstrate and help learners to develop a "repertoire of movement patterns" (Gomez & Gomez, 1984; 38) from which they can choose depending on the patient situation. For example, the instructor could teach learners how to perform a urinary catheterization first with a patient in a supine position and then with the patient in a side-lying position, using both straight catheters and indwelling catheters, placing the sterile field on the bed and then on the overbed table. Although this approach requires the learner to absorb more initially, the chances of transferring the skill successfully to the clinical setting would be improved.

Two recent studies have attempted to shed some light on this subject of teaching open and closed skills amid various environmental stimuli. Benjamin et al (1984) explored the effect of extraneous conversation on learning and transfer of the skill of intramuscular injection. Fifty beginning baccalaureate nursing students were divided into experimental and control groups. Both groups demonstrated the skill after having received cognitive information and some practice. During the student demonstrations, learners in the control group were instructed not to talk, and the instructor said nothing. During the demonstrations by the experimental group, the instructor talked about unrelated topics and attempted to involve the learner in the conversation. Student performance was rated at that time and later when the learner first gave an intramuscular injection during clinical experience. Analysis of data showed that the highest clinical performance scores were achieved significantly more frequently by learners in the experimental group. Five of them noted that they found the distracting conversation the most stressful aspect of the initial demonstration. The researchers concluded, however, that "perhaps the use of this stress-producing distractor at the time of mastery also helped students to perform well in the stressful environment of a clinical setting" (Benjamin et al, 1984; 112). This study provides some evidence that maintaining skills in the open mode as much as possible in the college laboratory may enhance performance in the real world.

The second study was reported in 1987 by Gomez and Gomez. They investigated practice conditions for the open skill of taking blood pressure readings. Sixty-three baccalaureate nursing students were randomly assigned to experimental and control groups. The control group practiced taking blood pressures in the college laboratory; the experimental group practiced on a gynecologic postpartum unit in a hospital. Evaluation of the skill was done the following day in a nursing home. The group that practiced in the hospital had higher indices of accuracy and confidence than the group that practiced in the laboratory. The implication of this study is that some skills might best be practiced in clinical settings.

Without further research evidence, the decision as to where to teach skills may have to depend on certain practical factors, such as laboratory versus clinical access, potential patient risks, costs, and available time. It may be that some skills, even open skills, can best be taught in the nursing lab and others in the clinical lab. Whatever location is chosen, the instructor retains the responsibility for structuring the best possible learning environment.

Providing Feedback

The next point in the skill-learning process where the instructor plays an important role is the phase of feedback and decision making. Feedback is necessary for learning to take place, but each learner should be allowed to benefit from intrinsic (internal) feedback before being given extrinsic (external) feedback. After finishing the skill performance, the learner should have a short time in which to sense whether his or her motor plan was appropriate and whether outcomes were achieved. In fact, guiding students to attend to intrinsic feedback is a way teachers can help them learn to learn.

After a learner has paid attention to intrinsic feedback, the teacher should offer extrinsic feedback. The instructor can discuss and confirm the person's intrinsic feedback, determine whether it was accurate, and give additional advice as needed. Although the teacher should give the learner time to assimilate the skill movements before giving feedback, the delay should not be too long. Research has confirmed that extrinsic feedback is most effective when no interfering activity occurs between the skill performance and the accompanying feedback (Gomez & Gomez, 1984). In general, the novice needs more extrinsic feedback than the person who is nearing competence. The person who does poorly obviously needs much more precise and extensive feedback than the person whose early attempts approximate what is desired.

The way in which feedback is given can also influence the learner's motivation to persevere. Harsh criticism can discourage learners rather than spur them to correct the performance on another try. On the other hand, inappropriate praise will mislead learners into thinking that they performed well and have mastered the skill.

Structuring Practice

The second stage of Gentile's model, fixation/diversification, also has important teaching implications. In this stage the general motor pattern is practiced and refined. The learner attempts to reach a certain level of skill. Closed skills lend themselves fairly quickly to fixation of the motor pattern acquired in stage one, but open skills require refinement of a diversity of motor patterns depending on environmental conditions.

The teacher's role in this last stage is to structure the practice conditions and continue to provide feedback that will enable the learner to reach the desired skill level. Practice is essential in order to fix the sequential order of movements in the person's memory. The amount of practice needed varies with the complexity of the skill. Practice enables the learner to become masterful at performing the skill smoothly, with greater control and less wasted time and motion.

Continued practice must be accompanied by feedback, or it will not result in improved skill levels. Recall the learning proposition from Chapter 2, "Sheer repetition without indications of improvement or any kind of reinforcement is a poor way to attempt to learn." When students practice, they should initially have a more skilled person with them who can provide extrinsic feedback, or they should periodically review audiovisuals of experts performing the skill. They could also review tapes of their own performance. If the teacher has helped the student learn how to evaluate intrinsic feedback, he or she will eventually be able to progress without any outside help.

Massed versus Distributed Practice   Timing and sequencing of skill practice have been studied by many researchers. The efficacy of massed practice (no rest periods) versus distributed practice (planned rest periods) and the relative length of practice versus rest periods has been the focus of most studies.

A classic study was conducted in 1930 by Lorge (cited in De-Cecco, 1968; 287). Three groups of students tried to learn to draw a figure while looking only at mirror images of what they were doing. The first group were required to practice 20 times with no rest periods (massed practice). The other two groups were given rest periods between practice trials (distributed practice). The rest periods for these two groups ranged from 1 minute between each of the 20 trials for the first group to 1-day rest periods between trials for the second group. The time it took to complete the figure on each trial was measured. The results showed a consistent difference between massed- and distributed-practice groups. Both groups using distributed practice performed about the same, completing the task in less time than the massed-practice group on every trial after the first. Lorge's experiment demonstrated the superiority of distributed practice but showed no difference resulting from varying the length of rest periods.

In 1946 Kientzle studied spaced (distributed) practice. Her subjects performed the task of printing the alphabet upside down. She looked at the effects of various lengths of rest periods on performance, which was measured by the number of letters written per trial. Each practice trial lasted 1 minute, and rest periods varied from 0 seconds to 7 days. She found that groups with distributed practice gained more than groups with massed practice, and the trend was for longer rest periods to show the greater gains. The greatest gains were made with rest periods between 0 and 10 seconds, but gains continued to increase up to rest periods of 45 seconds. This effect was limited, however: The group with 7 days' rest performed no better than the group with 45 seconds of rest.

Kimble and Bilodeau (1949) studied the effects of the lengths of both practice periods (10–30 seconds) and rest periods (10–30 seconds). The learning task was overturning cylindrical blocks in a large board. The researchers discovered that shorter rest periods were more productive, but longer work periods were even more important. They also acknowledged that length of the rest period depends on length of the practice period, and the lengths of both depend on the type of task.

Another researcher (Duncan, 1951) attempted to discover whether distributed practice was still superior when the total amount of massed practice surpassed the amount of distributed practice. He discovered that the subjects using distributed practice performed better even though they had only one-third as much practice as the massed-practice group.

In summary, research indicates that for motor skills, distributed practice is best, that practice must be long enough for the learner to make appreciable progress, and that rest periods must be short enough that forgetting does not present a problem (Garrison & Magoon, 1972; 355). The actual length of practice and rest periods will vary with the particular skill. Reinforcement must follow soon after each practice session.

Attention to Other Stimuli   After sufficient practice, the learner reaches the end of the fixation/diversification stage. He or she can then perform the skill correctly with ease and with little or no anxiety. It is not until reaching this point that the learner can adequately attend to other stimuli in the environment.

During the period of heightened anxiety and concentrated attention that comes with skill learning, the learner usually reacts only to stimuli related to the task. Other stimuli are stored in short-term memory until the learner is free to attend to them (Gudmundsen, 1975; 24). That is why teachers often accuse students of having tunnel vision. They say to the student, "You did very well with that catheterization, but you didn't talk to the patient while you were doing it." Instructors can't expect learners who are performing psychomotor tasks to conduct high-level conversations until they have learned the skill quite well. Simple explanations to the patient about the steps of the procedure can be built into skill learning, however, so that as the individual learns to perform certain sequential steps, he or she also learns at what points to give simple explanations to patients.

Whole Versus Part Learning

Teachers debate whether skills should be learned in their entirety or whether they should be broken into their component parts and taught in sections. Research on this topic is not entirely conclusive.

In 1952, Knapp and Dixon found that teaching the whole skill of juggling was superior to teaching it in parts. McGuigan and McCaslin (1955) found the whole method to be superior to the part method in teaching army recruits how to fire a rifle. Cox and Boren (1965) discovered part and whole methods to be equally effective.

When Naylor and Briggs (1963) looked at interactions between task complexity, task organization, and whole or progressive-part methods of training, they found that the part-training group exceeded the whole-training group on high-complexity, low-organization tasks.

Recent research in this area is lacking, but the consensus is that the part method is efficient for skills that are not difficult or not highly organized and for skills that are so extremely complex that practicing the whole skill is almost impossible. The whole method, on the other hand, is superior for skills of moderate difficulty in which the parts of the skill are highly organized and interdependent (DeCecco, 1968; 286; Gomez & Gomez, 1984; 37).

Translating these precepts into everyday examples reveals many of both types of skills in nursing. Skills that could be taught by the whole method might include assessment of vital signs, dressing change, nasogastric intubation, and specimen collection. The part method might be most effective in teaching such skills as intramuscular injection (first drawing up medication, then injection), tracheostomy care (first suctioning, then cleaning), setting up a new intravenous line (first bottle and tubing, then calculation and regulation), and urinary catheterization (first gloving, then setting up the sterile field, then insertion and drainage).

Teachers should analyze each psychomotor skill according to its level of difficulty and the degree of interdependence of its parts. It would then be fairly easy to determine which skills should be taught by which method. The experienced instructor also knows which skills learners have the most difficulty mastering. These skills can be analyzed to see whether they can be separated into component parts for teaching purposes.

Retention of Skill Learning

Compared to other kinds of learning, psychomotor skills are retained particularly well. One reason for this retention is the fact that psychomotor skills may be more meaningful to the learner than cognitive data. Also, people are more likely to retain learning that requires a total body effort and that entails extensive practice.

Research on motor skill retention indicates that perceptual-motor skills are well retained even after long periods without practice (Fleishman & Parker, 1962). The amount of retention is determined by the level of proficiency attained. Thus, a nursing student who had learned how to give injections and who had given two injections in the clinical area before dropping out of school might not recall the procedure a year later. But a student who had graduated and had extensive practice in giving injections and who left nursing for a few years would probably recall the skill easily upon returning to nursing practice.

Even if some loss of retention does occur over a period of time, a skill that was initially well learned can be quickly regained with minimal relearning.

The College Skills Laboratory

Although the nursing laboratory has fallen into relative disuse in some colleges, it is being revived in many of them. In light of what is known about learning open and closed skills, it might seem best for students to learn many psychomotor skills in clinical agencies than in a lab setting. However, that is not always possible or economically feasible.

In many geographic areas, clinical agencies are at a premium and must be used as places where students can integrate and synthesize their knowledge. Using them to teach learners basic psychomotor skills would be a waste of potential clinical experiences. Students could better learn at least the rudiments of the skills in the college laboratory and practice them to the point of mastery in the clinical setting.

Teaching basic skills in clinical agencies is also expensive, because novices require intense supervision if they are performing skills for the first time. One instructor can probably effectively teach and supervise only a few learners in such circumstances. If, however, learners develop basic competence in the college laboratory, faculty in the clinical area can more realistically handle groups of eight to ten.

Learners themselves usually welcome the opportunity to practice their skills in the college laboratory before having to implement them in the more anxiety-provoking and hectic clinical agency. The lab is seen as a relatively safe and nonthreatening setting where students can concentrate on learning before they have to focus on performing.

Uses of the Skills Laboratory

A college skills laboratory can be used in a number of ways. Certain structures and methods of functioning may be workable in some schools but not in others, depending on the type of program, size of faculty and student body, availability of media, and philosophy of the program.

The college laboratory may be used primarily as a place for independent learning. In this configuration, a great deal of preparation must be done by the faculty. Audiovisual hardware and software must be selected and readily available. Learners must be aware of which software they should use at certain points of the curriculum. They should also be directed to additional readings that provide theoretical background for the skill.

Haukenes and Halloran (1984) describe a college laboratory where self-instruction is the primary teaching method. Learners are provided with a psychomotor skills handbook containing all skills taught throughout the curriculum. Each skill in the book is accompanied by information about the objectives of the skill lesson, the required and suggested media and reading, the necessary practice equipment and its location, and skill-testing procedures. The learners proceed at their own pace, deciding when to visit the college lab, how much time to spend with audiovisuals and practice, and when to schedule written and performance tests. Laboratory instructors assist the students as necessary and monitor the testing procedures.

Extensive use of the college lab in this manner necessitates a sizable expenditure. Learners must have up-to-date supplies and equipment with which to practice. Still, this expenditure is offset by the fact that clinical faculty will be able to work with larger groups of learners if they have already developed skill competence.

It is essential to have adequate teaching staff in the laboratory. Learners who practice without any feedback can be wasting their time; they need a knowledgeable person available in the lab. Bauman, Cook and Larson (1981) describe a setup in which learners are assigned independent learning time in the college lab but are given a student partner. The partner system provides the learners with a "patient" and also with someone who can provide some feedback in the absence of an instructor.

The college laboratory can be used as an extension of the clinical area, with learners and faculty rotating through the lab during scheduled clinical time (Hallal & Welsh, 1984; Taylor & Cleveland, 1984). With this plan, clinical faculty bring their students to the college laboratory to work closely with them on skill learning. The instructor may demonstrate a skill or show audiovisuals to the entire clinical group and then work with small groups of learners as they practice the skill. Additional practice time may also be available to the learners. Competence testing is done by the clinical instructor or by the college laboratory instructor, if there is one. Use of this model requires careful scheduling of college lab time.'

The college laboratory can be used in a number of other creative ways as well. For example, Rutledge, Sweeney and Shelby (1983) formulated a means for students to apply their observation and assessment skills. A "patient's unit" within the college lab was set up with a mannequin and equipment, and at least 30 errors of nursing care were built into the situation. The errors were such things as a Foley drainage bag lying on the floor or a nasogastric tube taped incorrectly on the mannequin's face. Learners were brought into the unit for 5 minutes to observe for possible errors and then worked in small groups to suggest corrective interventions and rationale.

Duprey and Patten (1986) describe a skills relay game that was used to provide motivation for developing proficiency in psychomotor skills. Students learned the rudiments of certain skills and were given practice time. Then a relay race was held, with clinical groups acting as teams. One member of each team came forward and drew a card indicating which skill was to be performed. The skill was then carried out, and its accuracy was judged by a faculty member. Then a new member from each team drew a card. Each team received points for success in speed and accuracy. Learners evaluated the game favorably and said it encouraged them to practice and achieve skill competence.

Skill Demonstrations

Inherent in most of these lab scenarios are skill demonstrations. Demonstrations are often shown via audiovisual media, but audiovisuals of some skills may not be available, may be of poor quality, or may not show procedures in a way that will be expected of learners. Faculty then have to demonstrate skills to groups of students. New teachers sometimes find demonstrations to be anxiety provoking (sometimes veteran teachers do, too). Following are some guidelines for skill demonstrations that will make them less threatening and enhance their usefulness.

Careful preparation takes a lot of the uncertainties out of demonstrations. Well before the time of the demonstration, you should assemble all the necessary equipment. Besides ensuring that you have everything, make sure that it is all in working order. Nothing is more frustrating or embarrassing than finding that you have to improvise during a demonstration because some equipment is nonfunctional. Run through the procedure just as you will when the class is watching. Make sure that all of the learners will be able to hear you and see what you are doing. Keep track of how long the demonstration takes during the trial run.

Decide ahead of time whether you want the class to take notes. Note taking can distract the learners' attention from what you want them to see. If you don't want any note taking, make sure that explanatory information is in the textbook and refer the learners to it. You could also prepare a handout with all the important information and distribute it after the demonstration.

If feasible, you might videotape your demonstration. If the tape turns out well, you won't have to repeat any more live demonstrations unless you wish to do so. You could also have someone take slides of your demonstration and later narrate a tape to accompany it. Goldsmith (1984) researched the effectiveness of videotape versus slide-tape programs in teaching the skill of sterile dressing change and found both to be equally effective.

When you are ready for the actual demonstration, arrange for the environment to be as realistic as possible. Have all equipment nearby and ready for use. Perform the procedure step by step, explaining your actions as necessary and the rationale for each step. You might ask the class to answer questions about what you are doing and why, and what would happen if you did something differently, to keep them actively involved. You can ask students to assist you when needed. If there is more than one way to proceed, you can explain that as you go along. Go slowly enough that the group can follow all of your actions. During the performance, or at the end, you can ask for questions.

Whatever the skill you are demonstrating, be sure that you adhere to all of the principles of good nursing care. For example, always incorporate aseptic technique, good body mechanics, and patient privacy. Cutting corners because "it is just a demonstration" can mislead students into thinking that these things are not important for all situations.

Because there is no body of research indicating the most effective way to demonstrate skills, it might be wise to use several approaches in teaching a particular skill. Depending on available instructional tools, this could be done in a variety of ways. You could have learners watch an audiovisual that explains the whole procedure, then give a demonstration yourself in which you show the step-by-step progression but with minimal talking. Giving explanations during a demonstration might distract some learners' attention from the procedure being performed. You could also give a live demonstration with all of the explanations and then have the students watch a silent film loop of the skill. As another option, students could first read about the procedure and then have it demonstrated to them.

Mental Imagery

Mental imagery is a technique that has been widely studied and applied in physical education. The basic premise is that learners and performers can improve their skill level not only by physical practice but also by mental practice. A moving model of correct performance is implanted in the mind, and for some unclear reason this mental image of how the skill is to be performed helps to improve performance. Such mental practice might work by means of establishing habits in the neuromuscular system at a subliminal level. It is also possible that mental practice is strictly a cognitive phenomenon in which specific pathways of concentration are laid down in the mind or that a favorable mindset is established toward the skill (Start & Richardson, 1964).

After more than 50 years of use by other disciplines, nurse educators are starting to apply what is known about mental imagery (also known as mental practice, guided imagery, visual imagery, symbolic rehearsal, and imaginary practice) to teaching psychomotor skills in nursing. If the technique works well in learning psychomotor tasks in physical education, why not in nursing?

Research on Mental Imagery

Richardson (1967) reviewed some 25 studies on the ability of mental practice to improve motor skills such as tennis drives, basketball shots, juggling, card sorting, and ring throwing. He found 11 studies in which statistically significant results pointed toward the association of mental practice and improved performance on a task. Seven more studies showed a "positive trend" toward the

effectiveness of mental practice, and only three studies reported
negative findings. He also found evidence to suggest that alternating mental practice with physical practice is as good as or better
than physical practice alone.

Two other investigators focused on whether physical practice
is needed at all in learning certain skills; perhaps mental practice
would be enough. Jones (1965) found that his subjects successfully
performed a simple gymnastic skill using only mental practice as
preparation. Phipps and Morehouse (1969) discovered that while
mental practice alone was sufficient for performing the same simple
gymnastic skill that Jones used, mental practice alone was not
sufficient when the subjects had to learn a more complex skill.

Learners vary in their ability to conjure up and retain mental
images. Eaton and Evans carried out a study to determine whether
"nursing students who had low ability to form images could have
their imaging ability enhanced through the use of imaging exercises" (1986; 193). They found that after only two brief practice
sessions the abilities of subjects with previously low imagery were
significantly enhanced, and in fact these subjects surpassed the
high-imagery group.

Researchers have explored whether the ability to use and benefit from mental imagery is correlated with any other abilities. The
results of such studies have indicated a lack of relationship between mental imagery and intelligence, comprehension, abstract
thinking, logical thinking, mental multiplication, mechanical reasoning, sex, and school marks (Start & Richardson, 1964; Richardson,
1967).

Implementing Mental Imagery

To use the imagery process in teaching psychomotor skills, you
first have to analyze a skill and separate it into sequential steps, as
you do when teaching a skill by the demonstration method. Then
you have to combine the procedural steps with instructions on how
to implement mental practice. Full instructions should be written
out if you intend to have the students use the process at home.

When you are introducing the mental imagery method in the
classroom or college laboratory, you should follow a few basic
procedures. First, introduce the concept of mental imagery and
explain how it can be useful in learning psychomotor skills. Tell the
learners that you will be helping them mentally practice a skill that
they have already seen demonstrated (and one with which they

may already have had some physical practice). Stress that research indicates that for best results, mental practice should be alternated with physical practice.

Structure the environment to reduce distracting stimuli such as noise or bright lights. If the class has been boisterous prior to the time in which you want them to begin mental imagery, have them perform a few relaxation exercises first, such as taking deep breaths and consciously relaxing each limb.

Instruct the students to sit in a comfortable position and close their eyes. Closing the eyes is optional, because when practicing on their own the learners may have to read the instruction sheet; in a group session it is effective in helping the learners concentrate.

Begin the instructional practice sequence in a soft voice. A typical session for a simple skill like handwashing might go something like this:

1. Close your eyes.
2. Picture yourself standing in front of a sink. The sink has one spout and both hot and cold water faucets. There is a soap dispenser on the wall above the sink to the right. There is a paper towel dispenser above the sink to the left.
3. Imagine pushing your wristwatch a few inches up your wrist.
4. You are now turning on the hot and cold water faucets.
5. Adjust the water to a comfortable warm temperature.
6. Picture yourself rinsing your hands well in this warm water.
7. Leave the water running and with your right hand get some soap from the dispenser.
8. Imagine yourself spreading the soap over all surfaces of your hands. Your hands now feel slippery.
9. Rub each part of your hands. Start with your palms, then the backs of your hands, now each finger. Look to make sure that you have enough lather; if not, get more soap.
10. Picture yourself rinsing your hands, letting the water start at your fingertips and run off your wrists. Make sure no soap is left on your hands.
11. Let the water run while you reach with your left hand for a paper towel. Dry your hands briefly and use the damp towel to turn off the water.

12. Take another paper towel to dry your hands completely.

13. Throw the paper towel in the wastebasket.

14. Now return your attention to the classroom and open your eyes.

Explain to the class how often you expect them to use the mental practice procedure. Tell them that many athletes have found that using mental practice immediately before an important trial (similar to a skill test) helps them improve performance and reduce stress.

You may encounter a few difficulties in implementing mental imagery (Richardson et al, 1984). Initially some learners may not take the whole process seriously, and you may hear a few giggles and murmurs when their eyes are closed. After some experience with mental practice, when these same students realize that it is effective, they will take it more seriously. A few students may have difficulty concentrating on the imaginary skill; they may report that when they are alone their mind wanders. For these students, try having them first read the instructions and picture each step separately. Then, when they have channeled their thoughts, have them go through the whole process again with their eyes closed.

Summary of Research

Educators must continue to research and apply new techniques to teaching psychomotor skills. Although a lot of research has been done on psychomotor skills in other disciplines, many of the same types of studies must be done on nursing skills. Which skills should be taught in college laboratory versus clinical laboratory settings? Which skills could most effectively be taught by part versus whole methods? How can nurse educators most effectively demonstrate skills to groups of students? For which skills or which students does mental imagery work best? Can mental imagery reduce anxiety associated with learning complex nursing skills?

The studies that could flow from interest in psychomotor learning are almost limitless. In a practice discipline, clinical skills are numerous and consume a lot of learning time. Anything instructors can do to increase the efficiency and effectiveness of this learning time deserves investigation.

References

Bauman K, Cook J, Larson LK: Using technology to humanize instruction: an approach to teaching nursing skills. *J Nurs Educ* (Mar) 1981; 20:27–31.

Benjamin G et al: Use of extraneous conversation in the teaching of nursing skills. *J Nurs Educ* 1984; 23:109–113.

Cox JA, Boren LM: A study of backward chaining. *J Educ Psych* 1965; 56:270–274.

De Cecco JP: *The Psychology of Learning and Instruction.* Prentice-Hall, 1968.

Duncan CP: The effect of unequal amounts of practice on motor learning before and after rest. *J Exper Psych* 1951; 42:257–264.

Duprey MPC, Patten BC: Playing for proficiency: a new approach to motivation and psychomotor learning. *J Nurs Educ* 1986; 25:348–351.

Eaton SL, Evans SB: The effect of nonspecific imaging practice on the mental imagery ability of nursing students. *J Nurs Educ* 1986; 25:193–196.

Fleishman EA, Parker JF: Factors in the retention and relearning of perceptual-motor skills. *J Exper Psych* 1962; 64:215–226.

Garrison KC, Magoon RA: *Educational Psychology.* Charles E. Merrill, 1972.

Gentile AM: A working model of skill acquisition with application to teaching. *Quest* 1972; 17:3–23.

Goldsmith JW: Effect of learner variables, media attributes, and practice conditions on psychomotor task performance. *West J Nurs Res* 1984; 6:229–240.

Gomez GE, Gomez EA: The teaching of psychomotor skills in nursing. *Nurse Educator* (Winter) 1984; 9:35–39.

Gomez GE, Gomez EA: Learning of psychomotor skills: Laboratory versus patient care setting. *J Nurs Educ* 1987; 26:20–24.

Gudmundsen A: Teaching psychomotor skills. *J Nurs Educ* (Jan) 1975; 14:23–27.

Hallal JC, Welsh MD: Using the competency laboratory to learn psychomotor skills. *Nurse Educator* (Spring) 1984; 9:34–38.

Haukenes E, Halloran MCS: A second look at psychomotor skills. *Nurse Educator* (Autumn) 1984; 9:9–13.

Jones JG: Motor learning without demonstration of physical practice under two conditions of mental practice. *Res Quarterly* 1965; 36:270–276.

Kientzle MJ: Properties of learning curves under varied distributions of practice. *J Exper Psych* 1946; 36:187–211.

Kimble GA, Bilodeau EA: Work and rest as variables in cyclical motor learning. *J Exper Psych* 1949; 39:150–157.

Knapp CG, Dixon WR: Learning to juggle: a study of whole and part methods. *Res Quarterly* 1952; 23:398–401.

McGuigan FJ, MacCaslin EF: Whole and part methods in learning a perceptual-motor skill. *Amer J Psych* 1955; 68:658–661.

Naylor JC, Briggs G: Effects of task complexity and task organization on the relative efficiency of part and whole training methods. *J Exper Psych* 1963; 65:217–224.

Phipps SJ, Morehouse CA: Effects of mental practice on the acquisition of motor skills of varied difficulty. *Res Quarterly* 1969; 40:773–778.

Richardson A: Mental practice: a review and discussion. *Res Quarterly* 1967; 38:95–107.

Richardson GE et al: Educational imagery and the allied health educator. *J Allied Health* 1984; 13:38–47.

Rutledge DN, Sweeney J, Shelby J: The "situational": a new teaching-learning strategy for basic nursing skills. *Nurse Educator's Opportunities & Innovations* (May) 1983:2–3.

Start KB, Richardson A: Imagery and mental practice. *British J Educ Psych* 1964; 34:280–284.

Taylor JA, Cleveland PJ: Effective use of the learning laboratory. *J Nurs Educ* 1984; 23:32–34.

Chapter 9

Clinical Laboratory Teaching

Teaching in a clinical laboratory setting is so complex that few researchers have accepted the challenge to study the teaching and learning that take place there and how both can be improved. Without a research base to work from, instructors rely on traditional wisdom, experience, and trial-and-error tactics to guide their performance.

Purpose of the Clinical Laboratory

What kind of learning does take place in a clinical setting? What are the real purposes behind having learners spend time in clinical agencies? Some of the answers are apparent; some we can only guess at.

It seems obvious to expect theory and practice to come together in the clinical laboratory. Learners should have the opportunity to apply the theoretical concepts, rules, and propositions they have learned in the college classroom. A proposition like "Frequent change in body position helps prevent decubitus ulcers" can be tested with various patients to see how and under what conditions it holds true. Learners not only test the proposition but learn when to apply it, and they practice the techniques of implementation. The proposition becomes more than a memorized fact; it takes on life and meaning as it is applied to real patients. Students learn how this one piece of information fits into the whole picture of nursing in a more realistic way than they ever could in a classroom.

It is in the clinical laboratory that many skills are perfected. Complex psychomotor skills may be practiced initially in a college lab, but to be mastered, they often require a live rather than simulated situation. For example, learners can practice colostomy care endlessly in a simulation lab, but they will never become experts at it until they work with a variety of patients who have different stomas and different skin conditions and contours, using various equipment. Communication skills and assessment skills are similarly developed in a clinical setting (Windsor, 1987).

Infante (1985), in her study of the clinical laboratory, noted that the opportunity for observation is an essential element of the clinical laboratory. The skill of observation can be taught in simulated situations, but learners need repeated experience observing patients in varied circumstances so that they know what to look for in changing situations.

Problem-solving and decision-making skills are also refined in the clinical laboratory. Students should learn the basics of these cognitive skills in the classroom and should practice them in class and college laboratories as described in previous chapters. The ultimate practice in decision making and problem solving, however, is done in patient settings with many interacting variables and constantly changing circumstances. Learners need practice using these cognitive skills under the guidance of an educator and other professional staff in real-life settings.

Learners also gain organization and time management skills in clinical settings. Again, no simulation can prepare students as well as the live laboratory when it comes to organization. It is in real clinical practice, with help from the instructor, that students learn how to organize all the data that bombard them, all the requests made of them, and all the intellectual and psychomotor tasks they must perform. They learn to set priorities by having repeated practice in doing so in complex situations.

Finally, nursing students become professionally socialized in the clinical laboratory. They learn which behaviors and values are professionally acceptable or unacceptable. The knowledge and skills they have learned become integrated into a nursing role. They begin to see staff nurses as role models, and they have opportunities to interact with members of other disciplines on a professional level. Students also gradually learn how to relate to patients professionally. Part of socialization into the nursing role involves "developing a commitment to be responsible for one's own actions" (Reilly & Oermann, 1985; 80). This kind of professional obligation can best be learned and nurtured in clinical situations where consequences for one's actions are readily apparent and where accountability is demanded.

For all of these reasons, nursing students need to spend time in clinical settings, and faculty need to learn how best to use that time.

Misuse of the Clinical Laboratory

As Infante (1985) points out clearly, the clinical laboratory has historically been misused in many nursing programs at all levels of nursing education. Nursing students have been sent to the clinical setting to gain work experience rather than to achieve educational objectives. Novices have been given almost total responsibility for patient care and have been supervised rather than taught. This misuse of clinical experience continues today in many places.

Faculty must examine the way in which the clinical laboratory is being used. Clinical objectives should be as clear and specific as those for the classroom or college lab. Objectives for beginning learners should be quite limited, focusing on specific processes of care. It is unrealistic to expect learners in their first or second clinical course to provide total patient care. Such expectations lead to excessive student anxiety, instructor fatigue, and increased chance of errors. It is only after the various components of patient care have all been practiced that the learner is able to integrate previous learning and provide total care.

For example, if the first clinical course is one in which students learn assessment techniques, data collection, and basic nursing skills, these processes should be practiced in small segments in the clinical lab sessions. In one session the objective might be for the learners to collect and record a health history. Other sessions might include a focus on physical assessment of various body systems. Bedbaths and bedmaking or administration of medications might be the objectives for still another lab. Expecting students to practice all these skills on the same day is overwhelming even if they have practiced the skills in the college laboratory.

Learners who are further along in the curriculum and who have demonstrated competence in individual skills can be expected to put it all together and provide total care. Integration of knowledge represents high-level cognitive activity and is appropriate for upper-level students.

Faculty who talk about "supervising" students in the clinical laboratory may be revealing an unconscious attitude toward student activity. They may be expecting learners to "perform" rather than to "practice." A certain amount of supervision must take place, but the emphasis should be on teaching and guiding. Teachers should expect learners to make mistakes but must avoid setting them up to make mistakes. Learners should not be functioning

independently in situations with a high level of risk. They should
be providing care in circumstances for which they are well quali-
fied and for which they have had preliminary guidance. Then
supervision becomes less of a priority and teaching becomes a
greater priority (Infante, 1985).

Preparation for Clinical Instruction

To ensure a positive clinical learning experience for students, faculty must do a great deal of planning before a course begins.
Clinical sites must be selected and contract negotiations with the
chosen agencies must be completed. Orientation sessions have to
be scheduled. Finally, before each clinical session, assignments
must be planned for each learner.

Selection of clinical sites should be done methodically. Geographical location is often the first consideration. Careful consideration should be given to the commuting distance for both instructors and learners. Long distances mean wasted time and extra
expense.

Another factor to be considered is the learning experience available. Will it be possible to obtain clinical experiences that correlate
with theoretical content? Will learners have a variety of experiences?
Is there enough room around the nurses' station or office for learners
to use patients' charts? An often overlooked aspect of the learning
experience is the availability of role models for learners. What are
the educational credentials and experience levels of the staff, and
are they receptive to having learners in the agency? Also, is the staff
in agreement that the faculty member will be in control of the
learners' educational experience? All these factors are important.

Sometimes more than one clinical site is used in a course. This
arrangement may be necessary and desirable for a number of
reasons, but caution should be used in selecting multiple sites. In a
15-week semester, two sites may be satisfactory, but more than two
creates problems. Students lose learning time in being oriented to
multiple agencies, and their stress levels may be increased by the
frequent shifting around. Moving to different units within the
same agency is not quite as traumatic, because even though the
place and people change, the basic policies and procedures probably do not.

Contracts must be drawn up between the school and the clinical
agency. It is sometimes the instructor's role to conduct the prelim-

inary contract negotiations. Schools of nursing usually stipulate in the written contract that certain units will be available to faculty and learners on certain days at specified hours. The contract usually covers such requirements as parking facilities and conference and locker space. Cafeteria access may also be stipulated. The clinical agency usually requires that the contract include the student-faculty ratio, evidence of completion of health records for all students and faculty, and evidence of malpractice insurance for students and faculty. The type of orientation program available to or required of learners and faculty may also be a part of the contract.

In addition to negotiating with the agency's administration or education department, faculty should set up a meeting with the head nurse or supervisor of the unit being used. At that meeting, the expectations of both parties can be discussed and actual implementation of the learning experience can be worked out. This is the appropriate time to share the course and weekly clinical objectives with the head nurse. If the staff are familiar with the learning objectives, they can assist learners in meeting them.

Orientation sessions for faculty new to an agency are essential. The students' learning experience flows more smoothly if the instructor is familiar with agency policies and procedures and is acquainted with the staff. Orientation programs may be formal or informal and can last from a few hours to a few days.

Student orientation may be conducted by faculty or by agency staff. The breadth of the orientation depends on the agency and on the level of the student.

After all these arrangements have been made, faculty can proceed with final preparation for clinical instruction. This last step involves making specific assignments for learners on a weekly or daily basis. Staff input can be invaluable in planning assignments. Staff members usually know the patients and families better than the instructor does. If they are aware of the weekly objectives, they can direct the faculty member to suitable patients.

Goldenberg and Iwasiw conducted an investigation of the criteria used by faculty in selecting patients for students' clinical experience. Not surprisingly, the three most important criteria used in the selection process were "students' individual learning needs, patients' nursing care needs, and matching of patients' needs with students' learning needs" (1988; 260).

Assignments may be chosen by the faculty member, by faculty and learners together, or solely by learners, depending on the setting and scheduled availability of learners (McCoin & Jenkins, 1988; Treece, 1969). Involving learners in choosing patients for clinical experience helps assure assignments that meet individual learning needs and may reduce student anxiety. However, these advantages may be offset by the disadvantages of increasing learner workload and travel time.

Even if learners are not involved in choosing assignments, they may be held responsible for clinical preparation. A visit to the clinical agency may be required so that the learner can research the assigned patient's chart and meet the patient and family. Schools that do not require the learner to go to the agency prior to the clinical practice day may still expect preclinical planning. The arrangements in this case often involve the instructor gathering data from the chart and passing it on to the student. The learner is usually expected to research the medical diagnosis, lab tests, and medications and formulate possible nursing diagnoses and plans for intervention.

Conducting a Clinical Laboratory Session

After all the careful preparation by faculty and students, the clinical laboratory session begins. For many faculty, the day starts with a group preconference.

Preconference

During the preconference, planning of patient care continues. Learners usually share some of the results of their research from the previous day. Tentative nursing diagnoses are aired, and the assigned learner can discuss possible nursing interventions with the other students.

If time is available, all students can discuss their patients in some depth. If time is limited, and it usually is, the instructor might select just a few patients who typify the focus of the day's objectives. For example, if the objectives revolve around fluid and electrolyte problems, the teacher would have a student with a surgical patient discuss the patient's fluid balance and the accompanying nursing responsibilities. Another learner with a patient who has congestive heart failure could present the identified problems in that case. The other learners should be able to transfer some of the information to their own patients.

Preconference time may also be used to help learners organize their day and prioritize the care they must give. Arrangements can be made to supervise certain student activities throughout the day.

Wolf and O'Driscoll (1979) conducted a survey of 146 NLN-accredited baccalaureate nursing programs to gather information about the use of preclinical conferences. Although 77% of respondents reported that preconferences were not mandatory, 81% did hold them. The authors inferred from these data that faculty seem to find preclinical conferences useful. The respondents said that patient care was "always discussed" and that "student feelings, health team relationships, professional nursing behaviors, and moral, ethical, and legal issues were frequently dealt with" (p. 457). In relation to the process of learning, "respondents said that students frequently asked questions; identified specific problems; . . . drew conclusions about, suggested alternative approaches to, and determined priorities among problems; . . . applied summarized information to a specific issue" (p. 457).

The Practice Session

Following the preconference, the learners begin their practice for the day. The structure of the practice session may vary a great deal. For example, each learner may be providing some degree of care to one or more patients and may be reporting directly to the faculty member with all data, all questions, and all needs for help and supervision. In another type of structure, students may work closely with staff nurses who answer many routine questions and provide some supervision and assistance, while the instructor spends time with those learners who are in situations calling for intense teaching and guidance. It is also possible to structure preceptorships in which learners (or orientees) work closely with a staff nurse who is partially responsible for teaching them, while the instructor is primarily involved in planning, organizing, and evaluating learning.

Learners may also be double-assigned to patients. That is, for complex nursing care situations, two learners may be assigned to one patient. Each learner has a specific role and clearly defined responsibilities. This structure fits well with high-acuity patients and large numbers of students.

The way a clinical experience is structured may vary from course to course or instructor to instructor within one school, depending on course objectives, level of students, and available clinical facilities and staff.

A variety of teaching methods can be used during practice sessions. Teachers have long used combinations of demonstration, lecturing, questioning, and guided discovery techniques. Questioning and discovery learning in particular can be used to assist learners in developing problem-solving and decision-making skills. Nursing care plans are also standard teaching devices. All of these methods have been dealt with in previous chapters.

Observation assignments have also been used routinely. Learners are assigned to observe nurses or other professionals performing various aspects of health care that students usually cannot perform. Learners might be placed, for instance, in an open-heart recovery room for a few hours of observation. Given some guidelines that channel their observations, they can find this to be a valuable experience. If they can be paired off with individual nurses whom they can observe and question, the learning experience may be even better. Observation experiences can be overused, however. They should be assigned sparingly so that they do not jeopardize the time available for actual practice.

Another teaching device is the *process recording*, a strategy frequently used to help students develop their communication and relationship skills. Learners are asked to record conversations (either during or immediately after they take place) between themselves and their patients. The format may include:

patient comment

nurse's reply

accompanying nonverbal communication

interpretation of the interaction

suggestions for self-improvement

By analyzing their communication patterns and discussing them with faculty, learners can improve their professional interactions with patients.

Clinical logs or *journals* may also be assigned to meet certain learning objectives. The learner is asked to write brief notes about each clinical day. These notes may take various forms, depending on the objectives of the assignment. Some instructors may want learners to focus on what they actually did during a clinical session and to evaluate their nursing care. This approach is useful in cases where the instructor is not spending much time with each student or when immediate postconferences are impossible. Other instructors may ask learners to record their impressions and feelings about their clinical day in order to focus on affective learning. Written or oral feedback from the instructor regarding the information in the journal is essential if it is to serve as anything but busywork for the student.

A teaching method that some faculty and inservice instructors have used successfully is *nursing rounds*, in which a group of learners and their instructor visit patients to whom the students are assigned. Skurski (1985) describes a procedure in which the learners inform their patients that their classmates and instructor will be in for a brief visit. Before entering the room, the assigned student briefly informs the group about the patient and the diagnosis. Once in the room, the same learner interacts with the patient while the others observe as much as they can about the patient and environment. The instructor may point out the use of certain equipment or procedures. All other discussion occurs in the corridor after the visit. The nursing diagnoses and planned nursing care are explained by the assigned learner, and the other learners ask questions, share their observations, and contribute ideas about the patient's care.

The purpose of nursing rounds is to expose learners to more nursing situations and to encourage them to consult with each other in planning and evaluating nursing care. Nursing rounds provide many opportunities to apply classroom theory to patient situations and to compare and contrast the patient care. Postconferences become more meaningful when students have met many or all of the patients being discussed.

Carpenito and Duespohl (1981) express concern about the possible violation of patient rights when nursing rounds are conducted. Although patients are asked for permission for the group to visit, they may be afraid to say no even if they do not want a group to come in. The ethics of the situation must be of concern, but carefully working out the procedure so that discussion is minimal and a minimum of time is actually spent in the patient's room may reduce the inconvenience for patients.

Postconference

Discussions with educator colleagues over the years have confirmed my belief that clinical postconference is one of the most challenging educational arenas for nurse educators. The challenge arises from several sources. First, postconferences are often un-structured seminars that allow for creativity but that can dissolve into meaninglessness. Second, the conference is usually held at the end of a physically and emotionally draining practice session. Third, a few learners in each clinical group seem to believe that they learned everything that could be learned during their practice time and feel that a postconference is just a boring postmortem session.

Postconference time is an ideal opportunity for pointing out applications of theory to practice, for analyzing the outcome of hypothesis testing, and for evaluating nursing care. To make the most of the opportunity, the faculty member should have objectives in mind for the session.

The least creative use of the clinical postconference is simply having each learner report what was done for his or her patient. This may in fact be a waste of time, because the instructor probably already knows most of what went on, as do many of the other learners who have talked among themselves and helped each other during the lab session. Instead of having each learner report during this time, it would be preferable for postconferences to revolve around just one or two learners' experiences, with the other learn-ers asking questions and contributing to the discussion by compar-ing or contrasting their own experiences. Rotating the focus to different learners each week will keep everyone involved.

The primary topic for discussion should fit in with the lab objectives. If the purpose of the clinical lab is to gain experience with ways of promoting respiratory function, the postconference should revolve around that objective in some way. For instance, a learner who cared for a patient with postoperative atelectasis might be asked to describe the course of the hospitalization, the pa-thophysiology, and related routine nursing care. A profitable dis-cussion could then be opened to allow learners to think about why preventive care for atelectasis was not given or why it didn't work. They could be led to talk about the corrective care that was given and to evaluate its effectiveness. The instructor could channel the discussion to include information on the cost of this complication in terms of delayed recovery, prolonged hospitalization, and in-creased financial charges. Research on the effectiveness of preop-erative teaching would also be appropriate to the discussion.

Another way to handle the postconference might be to chal-lenge learners to intellectually defend the care they gave. The instructor might describe a particular patient and then say, "Kim, evaluate the care you gave to this patient in terms of how you helped to promote his respiratory function." Several learners could be asked a similar question about their assigned patients.

The same conference might include information on nursing techniques that were *not* used by the students. The instructor might make a summary statement like, "Some of you had experience today with giving nasal oxygen, in teaching coughing and deep breathing and observing chest physiotherapy. In your preparation for today, what other nursing techniques for promoting respiration did you read about, and why weren't they used for your patients?"

Postconferences, then, should primarily be an opportunity to think critically about the care that was or should have been given. They are an occasion for helping students relate classroom information to their particular patients. In addition, postconferences can be helpful in getting students to air their feelings about nursing in general or about their patients or clinical experience in particular. The postconference can also be used to socialize people into the world of nursing, to help foster professional attitudes and values.

Working with Agency Staff

While carrying out clinical practice during a laboratory session, the faculty member and learners are also working with the staff of the facility. The relationship established with staff can enhance or greatly detract from the learning experience. Nail and Singleton state their belief that

> in order for students to be assured of a positive learning experience, at least 80% of the nursing staff of a unit must actually prefer to have students. If the nurses on a unit merely tolerate students, then students should be assigned elsewhere. (1983; 21)

There is no doubt that a supportive staff is necessary. Even though the instructor retains the primary teaching responsibility, learners have to rely on staff to answer questions, to show them where to find certain equipment, to give or take reports about patients, and so on.

For staff to be interested in students' learning, they must be aware of the clinical objectives, the general philosophy of the educational program, and the instructor's teaching methods. If the instructor cannot meet formally with all of the staff prior to the first laboratory session, he or she should arrange short, informal sessions with as many staff members as possible. This personal approach, including showing an interest in individual staff members and in the working of the unit, will go a long way toward establishing a collaborative working climate.

Long-term relationships with staff on a unit are highly conducive to good learning experiences. If at all possible, faculty members should remain on the same clinical units from one semester to another. The atmosphere of trust and mutual respect that develops over time helps pave the way for positive learning conditions. Faculty learn which staff members can be relied on for help, which like to demonstrate skills to learners, and which have particular expertise that they might share with learners. The staff, in turn, learn that the instructor knows what he or she is talking about, that she is a skilled clinician, or that he values the knowledge of the staff people.

Faculty who pay attention to detail also enhance their relationships with agency staff. Posting assignments where all staff can see them before making out their own assignments for the day is a courtesy that should be observed. If any last-minute changes are made in the assignment, the involved staff members should be notified at once. Reminder stickers may be placed on charts or in Kardexes to indicate students' patients. Asking staff at the end of the day whether there were any problems involving learners and making last-minute rounds to ensure that learners remembered to fulfill all of their responsibilities help make the clinical experience a good one for all concerned.

Evaluating Student Progress

Clinical evaluation of students has been studied little, written about extensively, and talked about excessively. In spite of all the attention given to the subject, evaluation remains a difficult, subjective, time-consuming, and often puzzling chore. It is usually the least favorite task of nurse educators, yet it is inescapable.

Learners in the clinical area need the feedback and judgment of their work that evaluation gives them. They need to know how they are doing at one level before progressing to the next. Faculty must evaluate learners to determine how well they are meeting objectives and to certify that they are safe practitioners.

Nurse educators should keep in mind that no one has yet devised a way to render totally objective judgments about people's behavior. However, a lot is known about evaluation principles and practices. This knowledge helps to demystify the clinical evaluation process and to make it more scientific and perhaps less distressing.

Choices to Be Made Regarding Evaluation

Before beginning the process of evaluation, the individual teacher or the faculty as a group must make several philosophical and practical choices: Should the evaluation be formative or summative? Should it be norm referenced or criterion referenced? What type of grading system should be used?

Formative and Summative Evaluation   *Formative* evaluation is the ongoing feedback given to the learner throughout the semester. This continuing evaluation process helps the learner identify strengths and weaknesses and meet the objectives of the course efficiently. It prevents learners from being surprised at the end of the course with a judgment about their performance for which they were not prepared. Formative evaluation may be graded or nongraded.

Summative evaluation, as it sounds, is a summary evaluation given at the end of a course or unit. The purpose is to assess whether the learner has achieved the objectives and is ready to move on to the next experience. Summative evaluation results in a grade of some type being given.

Clinical evaluation in nursing almost always involves summative evaluation. It may also include formative evaluation, whether formal or informal. The wise nursing instructor provides formative feedback even if it is not required by the school. Students have a right to know how they are progressing in their clinical work, and faculty can protect themselves against charges that they violated due process of law if they can prove that a learner was kept apprised of clinical progress or lack of it. The evaluative information may be given on an incident-by-incident basis, daily, or weekly. Surely learners should receive some information about their practice at least every 2 weeks.

Formative feedback may be given orally or in writing. If it is given orally, the instructor should also keep notes about what transpired. Written feedback is often more valuable because the learner can take time to read and absorb the information and the faculty member can keep a copy for future reference.

Written formative evaluation notes are often called *anecdotal records* or *clinical progress notes*. Rines (1963) advocated using anecdotal records to keep track of trends in student behavior. She specified that notes be written in two separate parts, a description of the observed behavior and the instructor's estimate of that behavior. Such notes can be jotted down on a file card after the clinical experience and shared with the student soon thereafter. Schuster and Colvin (1986) initiated a formal tool for writing clinical progress notes that incorporated information about the student assignment, the rationale for the assignment, observations related to student behavior, and evaluation of student progress.

Keeping detailed weekly records of students' clinical experience is time consuming, yet without such data, formative or summative evaluation is dependent on the instructor's memory, a fallible tool at best. Lacking such written documentation, the instructor who is called on to justify a final grade is on shaky ground.

Norm-Referenced and Criterion-Referenced Evaluation In *norm-referenced* evaluation, a student is compared with a reference group of learners, either those in the same class or in a norm group. Grading is therefore relative to the performance of the group. An evaluation process in which a student's behavior is characterized as "below average," "average," or "above average" or in which grades are distributed on a normal curve is norm referenced (see Figure 9-1).

Figure 9-1   **Example of Norm-Referenced Evaluation Items**

	Below Average	Average	Above Average
	(1 point)	(2 points)	(3 points)
1. Communicates therapeutically with patients			
2. Provides appropriate explanations to families of patients			

A number of problems are involved in using the norm-referenced system. Unless the evaluation tool is specific about what "average" behaviors are like, the process may be unreliable. One teacher's idea of average performance may be vastly different from another teacher's. If learners are compared to others in their clinical group, other problems arise. If every student in the group suffers from a poor level of performance, should all still receive a distribution of A's, B's, and C's simply because some are better or worse than others? When the standard of behavior is the peer group, such problems can become real.

Popham defines *criterion-referenced* evaluation as that "used to ascertain an individual's status with respect to a well-defined behavioral domain" (1978; 93). Krumme explains further that in criterion-referenced evaluation a person is "judged purely on whether or not she has met the performance criteria" regardless of how other students perform (1975; 766). Theoretically, in this system all students could earn A grades if they met a high standard of performance.

Criterion-referenced evaluation has been more popular in the past decade than norm-referenced evaluation (Pavlish, 1987; Reilly & Oermann, 1985; Sommerfeld & Accola, 1978). Many faculty believe criterion-referenced evaluation to be the fairer of the two types. Students are informed of the behaviors expected of them in order to pass or achieve a certain grade, and they either attain that level of performance or not (see Figure 9-2). Grading is less subjective when criteria are spelled out and each learner is held to that standard.

Figure 9-2   Example of a Criterion-Referenced Evaluation Item

Points

1. Communicates therapeutically with patients
    (Select one):

    a.   Communicates only when absolutely necessary. Informa-   (1)
         tion provided is sometimes inaccurate. Does not engage
         in active listening.

    b.   Communicates on a social level. Information given is   (2)
         accurate. Actively listens to patient concerns.

    c.   Actively listens and responds to patient concerns in a   (3)
         professionally helpful and accurate way.

In working with a variety of faculty and supervisory groups, I have found that clinical evaluation is often a mixture of both norm- and criterion-referenced approaches. Criteria for acceptable performance may be listed, but before making a final judgment about the grade, the instructor mentally compares the learner to others in the class. This comparison may result in a change in grade. For example, Sharon Smith seems to meet all the behavioral criteria for a B grade. But I have just given a B to Sam Jones, and I think that Smith should not receive as high a grade as Jones because of some subtle and not so subtle differences in their performance. So, I go back and reduce Smith's grade to a B–. Some faculty think this kind of flexibility in evaluation is justifiable and necessary; others view it as a travesty of the whole system of criterion-referenced evaluation.

Grading Systems   The issue of grading also enters the picture when choices are being made about various systems of evaluation. The two most common options for grading are assigning letter grades and using a pass/fail or satisfactory/unsatisfactory approach. Many schools require that letter grades be given in all courses, so instructors are forced to arrive at letter grades whether they are using norm-referenced or criterion-referenced methods.

Rines strongly asserted that clinical grades always be given on a pass/fail basis since "human behavior of any description is much too complex to permit such fine discriminations" as required in assigning numerical or letter grades (1963; 17). Many educators have been influenced by Rines's work and agree that letter grades are impractical and unfair when judgments about behavior are involved.

Criterion-referenced evaluation especially lends itself to the pass/fail system. Criteria describing minimally acceptable behaviors can be written, and the learner either performs at that level or does not. The teacher does not have to agonize over several gradations of behavior.

Faculty who work in schools that require letter grades have found ways to incorporate pass/fail clinical grading into the system. A common method used when theory and clinical practice are combined in one course is to give letter grades for the theory portion of the course and pass/fail for the clinical component. The total course grade is the theory grade as long as the student receives a pass for clinical work. If the learner fails the clinical portion, a failing grade is given for the course regardless of the theory grade earned.

Another issue to be considered is the point when students should be graded for clinical work. Teachers should be clear about when they are teaching and when they are formally evaluating and grading performance. Litwack, Linc & Bower identify the problem:

> ... students are often placed in a no-win situation: faculty members tell students that the practice setting or model lab is for learning and demonstration, but they may later use observations made and data gathered during the prac- tice time to determine, at least partially, students' grades and status. (1985; 9)

In many schools and clinical courses this exact situation exists. Anecdotal data collected in the second week of the semester may find their way into the final evaluation. There is no clear-cut evalu- ation period.

The most dramatic way to cure this problem is to institute an end-of-semester or end-of-level performance examination. Mor- gan, Luke & Herbert (1979) describe such a process. The New York Regents College Examinations also offer a performance evaluation system. The general idea is to set aside a few days at the end of the semester for clinical evaluation. Learners are placed in structured clinical situations for which they are given time to prepare, and they are evaluated as they provide specified aspects of patient care. Some of the evaluation may also take place in simulated situations in a college laboratory. These types of evaluation require substan- tial blocks of time and extensive scheduling.

If an end-of-course evaluation period is not feasible, some other means must be found to separate teaching/learning time from evaluation/grading time. At the very least, the first half of the clinical experience should be strictly learning time, and the last half would then produce data that contribute to the final grade. Non- graded formative evaluation can go on throughout the entire se- mester so that learners are aware of how well they are doing.

Behaviors to Be Evaluated

The components of clinical evaluation tools vary from one school to another and may differ for each clinical specialty. Nevertheless, certain basic ingredients appear in most evaluation tools. Evalu- ation occurs in three broad categories: the cognitive, psychomotor, and affective.

Rines (1963) claimed that most nursing faculty are concerned with evaluating four types of behaviors: implementation of nursing skills, appropriateness of judgment used in selecting approaches to help individual patients, ability to collect data from and give information to patients, and quality of relationships established with patients. Indeed, these four behavior groups do appear in some form in most of the tools that appear in the literature.

More specifically, the following learner behaviors are commonly evaluated by faculty:

observation and data collection

formulation of nursing diagnoses

goal setting

selection of nursing interventions

knowledge of rationale for interventions

psychomotor skills

evaluation of patient care

patient and family teaching

therapeutic communication

written documentation

organization of care

maintenance of patient safety

learner ethical behavior

learner initiative and responsibility

These behaviors are often categorized according to the nursing process (Cottrell et al, 1986; Cronin-Stubbs & Mathews, 1982; Hillegas & Valentine, 1986; Sommerfeld & Accola, 1978).

Evaluation Tools

The instrument or tool used for clinical evaluation should meet the following specifications:

1. The items should derive from the course or unit objectives.

2. The items must be measurable in some way. It must be possible to collect substantiating data.

3. The items and instructions for use should be clear to all who must use the tool.

4. The tool should be practical in design and length.

5. The tool must be valid and reliable. (Carpenito & Duespohl, 1981)

Few clinical evaluation tools in use today have been formally tested for validity or reliability. Therefore faculty are not sure that instruments are measuring what they want to measure, and they aren't certain that the outcome would be the same if different teachers used the tool to evaluate the same learner.

Both checklists and rating scales are appropriate tools for clinical evaluation. Checklists are usually used for summative criterion-referenced evaluation. The instructor often completes several checklists for each student, encompassing the major skills involved in the course. Thus, there may be checklists for psychomotor skills, communication skills, or written documentation. Each list includes specific behaviors that are checked by the instructor as being performed satisfactorily or unsatisfactorily. Some behaviors on the list may be considered critical; they must be performed satisfactorily or a failing grade will be given for the entire skill (see Figure 9-3).

Figure 9-3   **Checklist for Indwelling Catheter Maintenance (Urinary or Intravenous)**

Behavior	Satisfactory	Unsatisfactory
1. Checks for specific medical/nursing orders		
2. Maintains a closed system		
3. Maintains asepsis if system must be entered*		
4. Assesses patency every hour*		
5. Assesses insertion site appropriately		
6. Provides hygiene at insertion site		
7. Positions bag and tubing to facilitate flow		
8. Provides information/explanations for patient*		
9. Maintains accurate record of intake or output		

*critical elements

The exclusive use of checklists for summative evaluation re-duces the measurement of affective behaviors. For example, ethical behavior, responsibility, and initiative cannot be evaluated effec-tively by checklists. Some educators attack this problem by adopt-ing overriding statements about the necessity for students to be-have in an ethical and responsible manner in order to receive a passing grade.

Rating scales are used for both formative and summative and norm- or criterion-referenced evaluation. Rating scales consist of the behaviors to be evaluated and a graduated scale of measure-ment used to indicate the degree of skill or achievement that has been demonstrated by the learner (see Figures 9-1 and 9-2). The measurement scales can be written in terms of letter grades, points, or descriptors like "excellent, good, fair, poor" or "always, usually, sometimes, never" (Reilly & Oermann, 1985).

A weakness of the rating-scale approach is that teachers must each decide what constitutes an A level behavior or what "fair" or "usually" means. Some faculties develop written guidelines that help to differentiate among the gradations.

Sources of Evaluation Data

Information about student behavior comes from sources other than just faculty observation. Direct observation by instructors produces most of the data, but other sources should be used to give a bal-anced picture of performance.

Patients who have been cared for by the student can be asked some broad questions that will elicit data—for example, "How was your day, Mrs. C?" or "Is there anything else the student could have done for you, Mr. R?" It is helpful to validate this input with the learner to get both perceptions of the behaviors.

Learner self-evaluation data should be collected, especially from upper-level students. Self-evaluation is never an easy task, and learners must be taught how to do it. A survey by Abbott et al (1988) revealed that both students and faculty in one diploma program believed self-evaluation to be important. However, learn-ers felt that it was a more threatening experience than the instructor's clinical evaluation. Learners may evaluate themselves on the same tool as that used by the instructor, or they may provide their data in a personal interview or by means of a diary or log.

Data may also be gathered from agency staff. Formal evalu-ation is seldom sought from staff members unless they are serving as preceptors. Informal input, however, can be valuable because the staff may see the learner functioning in situations when the faculty member is absent. This information, good and bad, can also be shared with the learner.

Finally, written work submitted by the learner can be evaluated as part of the clinical grade. Nursing care plans, teaching plans, process recordings, and reports of observational experiences can all be used as clinical evaluation data as long as they meet the objectives of the clinical course.

Faculty-Student Conferences

All of the evaluative data that are collected, either on a formative or summative basis, should be shared orally or in writing with the student. Conferences should be held with the learner at least at midterm and for the final evaluation. The content of the conference is usually based on the information in the anecdotal records and the rating scales or checklists that are used. Positive feedback must be given along with the negative. Specific behaviors and critical incidents that are highly indicative of the learner's typical performance should be pointed out. The more specific and concrete the instructor can be, the more the learner will benefit from the evaluation. For instance, negative information may be given in two ways:

1. Jennifer, you have great difficulty implementing the nursing process. You need to develop skill in selecting nursing interventions for your patients.

2. Jennifer, in planning care for your patients, you have had difficulty in selecting the appropriate interventions that meet their specific needs. For example, when you cared for Paul, the 10-year-old with cerebral palsy, you tried to involve him in a game that was inappropriate for someone with his disability.

The second example provides better feedback for the student. The more specific examples a teacher can give to back up a generalization, the more the learner will understand and the less likely the teacher will be accused of being unfair.

If a learner is doing poorly, the teacher should call him or her in for frequent conferences and keep a record of those conferences. In addition to pointing out strengths and weaknesses, the instructor should work with the learner to develop a plan for improvement.

Learners who finally do fail the summative evaluation need a great deal of support. It must be made clear to them why they have failed. The failure then has to be put in perspective. Does it mean that the learner just needs more time and can retake the course? Or does it demonstrate that the learner lacks the ability to succeed in a nursing career? At some point in the conference, the learner's strengths and abilities should be emphasized to help the person regain a true picture of himself or herself.

Student Grievances Regarding Evaluation

Students in our society have the right to dispute a course or clinical grade. More and more students are bringing complaints against faculty members, including nursing faculty. In nursing education, most complaints involve clinical laboratory grades because they are the most subjective and the most difficult to explain to a learner who is doing poorly. However, faculty also have rights in the grading and grievance process, and means are available to help educators avoid litigation and protect them if litigation becomes inevitable.

The chief precaution that faculty can take is to ensure that students' rights to due process have been protected. This entails informing students of the course requirements, of their responsibilities, and of their progress in the course. It definitely means that faculty must keep records about each student's progress. The following list encompasses actions that faculty members can take to protect themselves and their students (Adams et al, 1979; Litwack, Linc & Bower, 1985; Majorowicz, 1986):

1. Distribute the academic standards policies and grievances policies of the school.

2. Distribute course requirements.

3. List the criteria for successful clinical performance.

4. Explain, in writing, how clinical grades will be derived.

5. Describe the consequences of receiving a failing clinical grade.

6. Keep anecdotal records of student experiences and performance.

7. Meet periodically with students to review performance and document these conferences.

8. Provide sufficient data on written evaluations to substantiate grades given.

9. If difficulties are encountered with a student, consult colleagues and department chairperson and document the consultation.

10. If a grievance is filed, follow the grievance procedure exactly as written.

11. Keep all records of student clinical performance until the student graduates.

Although teachers cannot always prevent grievances from being filed, they can reduce or eliminate the possibility of having a grade changed or a decision reversed if they follow these guidelines carefully and act in a reasonable and noncapricious manner toward students. The courts have not yet involved themselves in weighing the appropriateness of faculty decisions about student grades and clinical evaluations; they do, however, demand proof that the student was granted due process (Litwack, Linc & Bower, 1985).

Being accused of unfairness or ill will toward a student is an unpleasant experience and is upsetting to most faculty, but it is inevitable for teachers who stay in education long enough. The knowledge that one has done everything possible to protect students' rights and to provide a fair evaluation of their achievements goes a long way toward helping a teacher preserve a sense of proportion and confidence.

Working with learners in the clinical laboratory is a hectic, demanding, and sometimes anxiety-producing experience. Yet, it is also the aspect of teaching that often brings the greatest satisfaction and reward.

Research on Clinical Laboratory Teaching

It is not surprising that little research on clinical teaching has been conducted. The dynamics of learning in the clinical laboratory are complex. Many variables are operating in this setting, and research access is often limited. Yet the difficulties surrounding such investigations should not preclude attempts to learn more about how the clinical laboratory can best be used.

There are so many questions to be answered. How much structure and control in clinical assignments is beneficial? What is the optimum student-faculty ratio under varying conditions? To what degree do students learn from staff nurses? What aspects of socialization take place in the clinical area? What do learners actually gain from observational experiences? Does periodic written feedback have greater value than oral feedback? What are common sources of student grievances? Answers to these and similar questions would help establish a stronger scientific base for the teaching and learning that take place in clinical settings.

References

Abbott SD et al: Self-evaluation and its relationship to clinical evaluation. *J Nurs Educ* 1988; 27:219–224.

Adams E et al: Legal considerations in evaluating the clinical performance of students. *Considerations in Clinical Evaluation: Instructors, Students, Legal Issues, Data.* NLN Pub. No. 16-1764. 1979; 35–40.

Carpenito LJ, Duespohl TA: *A Guide for Effective Clinical Instruction.* Nursing Resources, 1981.

Cottrell BH et al: A clinical evaluation tool for nursing students based on the nursing process. *J Nurs Educ* 1986; 25:270–274.

Cronin-Stubbs D, Mathews JJ: A clinical performance evaluation tool for a process-oriented nursing curriculum. *Nurse Educator* (July/Aug) 1982; 7:24–29.

Goldenberg D, Iwasiw CL: Criteria used for patient selection for nursing students' hospital clinical experience. *J Nurs Educ* 1988; 27:258–265.

Hillegas KB, Valentine S: Development and evaluation of a summative clinical grading tool. *J Nurs Educ* 1986; 25:218–220.

Infante MS: *The Clinical Laboratory in Nursing Education,* 2d ed. Wiley, 1985.

Krumme US: The case for criterion-referenced measurement. *Nurs Outlook* 1975; 23:764–770.

Litwack L, Linc L, Bower D: *Evaluation in Nursing: Principles and Practices.* NLN Pub. No. 15-1976, 1985.

Majorowicz K: Clinical grades and the grievance process. *Nurse Educator* (March/April) 1986; 11:36–40.

McCoin DW, Jenkins PC: Methods of assignment for preplanning activities (advance student preparation) for the clinical experience. *J Nurs Educ* 1988; 27:85–87.

Morgan B, Luke C, Herbert J: Evaluating clinical proficiency. *Nurs Outlook* 1979; 27:540–544.

Nail FC, Singleton EK: Providing experiences for student nurses: perspectives for cooperating hospitals. *J Nurs Admin* (July/Aug) 1983; 13:20–26.

Pavlish C: A model for clinical performance evaluation. *J Nurs Educ* 1987; 26:338–339.

Popham WJ: *Criterion-Referenced Measurement*. Prentice-Hall, 1978.

Reilly DE, Oermann MH: *The Clinical Field: Its Use in Nursing Education*. Appleton-Century-Crofts, 1985.

Rines AR: *Evaluating Student Progress in Learning the Practice of Nursing*. Nursing Education Monograph. Teachers College, Columbia University, 1963.

Schuster SE, Colvin MK: Clinical progress notes: a challenge for the nurse educator. *J Nurs Educ* 1986; 25:33–36.

Skurski Sr V: Interactive clinical conferences: nursing rounds and education imagery. *J Nurs Educ* 1985; 24:166–168.

Sommerfeld DP, Accola KM: Evaluating students' performance. *Nurs Outlook* 1978; 26:432–436.

Treece EM: Students' opinions concerning patient selection for clinical practice. *J Nurs Educ* 1969; 8:17–25.

Windsor A: Nursing students' perceptions of clinical experience. *J Nurs Educ* 1987; 26:150–154.

Wolf ZR, O'Driscoll RW: How useful is the preclinical conference? *Nurs Outlook* 1979; 27:455–457.

PART

III

TECHNOLOGIES

Chapter 10

Audiovisual Technology in the Classroom

If used appropriately, audiovisuals and other technological methods can greatly enhance teaching and can add interest and stimulation to the classroom. If used inappropriately, these methodologies simply become time fillers and entertainers, serving no real educational purpose. A broad range of audiovisuals can be used effectively in the classroom, from pictures and charts to films and slides, complex computer programs and interactive videodiscs. It is important for the teacher to know what media are available, how to select them, how to use them effectively, and how to evaluate their use.

Why should one bother with technological methods of teaching? After all, it takes time to find good software, it takes energy to drag hardware around, the equipment all costs a lot of money, and just when everything is ready to go something breaks down and the teacher ends up lecturing anyway. Audiovisuals are nice, but they can be more trouble than they are worth. This is the (often hidden) attitude of many educators. But the fact remains that technologies can help instructors teach some things that they would not otherwise be able to teach at all, or would take much more time to teach, or would not be able to teach as effectively. For example, teaching learners how to make decisions in emergency situations can be done much more effectively and safely in a classroom using audiovisual or computer simulations than in a clinical setting. Medical terminology can be learned faster and in more interesting ways through technologies than through a teacher's lectures. Problem solving can be enhanced through audiovisual simulations, attitudes can be shaped when students are caught up in a vicarious visual world, and very important, retention and transfer can be maximized.

Selecting Media

How does an instructor begin to select the appropriate media and how and when should they be used? These decisions are based on a number of factors. The chief determinants are the course and class objectives. Some objectives may best be met by using lectures, some by role playing, some by individual student assignments, and some through the technologies. If several methods would be suitable, it may be best to opt for variety. A teacher may think that lecture/discussion would suit a particular unit of study very well even though media could also be used effectively. In this case, the lecture/discussions could be broken up with some media to provide interest and stimulation. Technologies should never be used simply because they fill time or make it easier for the teacher to entertain the students, but if the educational objectives can be met in an entertaining way, why not take advantage? After all, education can also be fun.

Let us see how a teacher might make a decision about use of media based on course objectives. Suppose that a nursing instructor has to teach a 4-hour unit on diabetes mellitus and related nursing care. The objectives for this unit are

> The student will:
>
> 1. explain the pathophysiology of diabetes.
> 2. identify assessments that should be made on the diabetic patient.
> 3. write a teaching plan for a newly diagnosed Type II diabetic.
> 4. evaluate the nursing care provided for a diabetic patient.

The teacher decides to lecture about the pathophysiology using overhead transparencies to explain the pathologic chain of events. Assessment could be taught by means of lecture, but the instructor decides to hold the students responsible for reading the material in the textbook and then shows slides illustrating some of the abnormalities that may be discovered on assessment of the diabetic patient. Because the class has 50 students, the instructor decides that it would be impossible to assist each student in writing a teaching plan, so students are asked as a group to contribute to a teaching plan while it is being written on an overhead transparency. Finally, the instructor decides to show a videotape of a nurse who is caring for a diabetic patient recovering from ketoacidosis and plans to have the students evaluate the care given by the nurse. With this mix of teaching methods all of the objectives can be met—and met more effectively and more interestingly than would be possible without technology.

Another factor to consider in deciding on media use is availability of both materials and technical assistance. What hardware (AV equipment) and software (AV programs) are available in the school or hospital? Is suitable material already there, or will it have to be purchased or rented? Does the school or hospital have a media staff or production specialist? Will the teacher have to learn how to operate equipment, or will someone else be able to run it? Is there someone to help make software, or will it have to be purchased? The answers to these questions will help in decisions on media use.

The level, ability, and number of students are important considerations in making decisions. Have students already had computer courses so they will know how to use the program assigned by the teacher? How motivated are the students to use audiovisual equipment on an individual basis? Is it too large a group to make individual media use feasible?

The level of the material being presented in the software must be evaluated. The complexity of the information and format should be suitable to college-level students or to practicing nurses. Material that is too simplistic—for example, health films designed for the general public—may not teach the professional very much. On the other hand, media designed for medical school use may require background knowledge that the students or nurses simply do not have.

The subject matter of the software must be up-to-date. If the material is not current, it is misleading to the students. Rental of software is preferable to purchase if the subject matter changes rapidly and will soon be out of date.

Reading catalogue descriptions of software is no substitute for actually seeing the product. An instructor should be careful about purchasing software without previewing it and never use software in class or assign students to use it without having seen or used it. Valuable learning time can be wasted if unsuitable software is not weeded out ahead of time.

Audiovisual Media

The most commonly used audiovisual media are handouts, chalkboards, overhead transparencies, slides, sound filmstrips, audiotapes, videotapes, and films. This section examines each, including how it can best be used, what its advantages and disadvantages are, and, in some cases, how to produce the software. Pertinent research findings are also included.

Handouts

Printed materials or handouts have been around for a long time and can be used to communicate facts, figures, and concepts. It may save a lot of time to give information in handout form rather than spend class time lecturing on it. Handouts are useful in supplying information unavailable in textbooks or by other media. If they are given out before a given class, they can be reviewed by students in preparation for class discussion. Printed materials also ensure that all students have access to the same information and can review that information whenever necessary.

Siegel's (1973) research indicated that printed lecture notes can enhance learning because the students receive all of the information without having to rely on in-class note-taking skills. MacManaway (1968) studied learning from lectures versus lecture scripts (handouts) and found that the scripts, especially when combined with small-group discussions, were at least as effective as live lectures, if not more effective. So handouts can be used to good purpose and can increase learning. However, a teacher should not rely so heavily on handouts that students cannot possibly read the mass of material given out.

Handouts should never be repetitious of the material provided in the textbook or given in live lectures. Discussions can profitably ensue from handouts, but a teacher should never waste in-class time reading all the information on the handout.

To be used effectively, handouts should be carefully planned. Necessary information should be typed neatly and concisely. Tables and charts are often useful for portraying information clearly. The teacher should explain the purpose of the handout and how it should be used. Unless handouts are going to be referred to during a class session, it is best to distribute them at the end of the period to prevent distraction during class. Printed materials given out at

the end of one class session can be used to whet the students'
appetites for the next.

Teachers may prepare their own materials and copy them on a
photocopier, spirit duplicator, or ink duplicator, or they may use
handouts available from various agencies or organizations such as
the American Heart Association, the American Diabetes Association, or the U.S. Department of Health and Human Services. The
wide variety of printed materials available are not all useful in
meeting course objectives, and unless the teacher selects them
carefully and plans how to use them, students may very well
ignore them.

Chalkboards

Chalkboards, blackboards, and the newer white felt-tip pen boards
are universally used in education and may never be replaced.
Although they have several uses, their outstanding feature is that
they allow for spontaneity in the classroom. New ideas or solutions
to problems can be jotted down as they are mentioned. If students
are suddenly confused about something, the point can be illustrated on the board. If students cannot visualize an object, it can be
quickly sketched. Chalkboards are especially useful for working
out mathematical problems, for outlining the material to be covered in class, and for having several students placing their ideas on
the board at the same time. Creative use of the chalkboard can add
dimension to almost any class.

To be used properly, a chalkboard must be placed where the
entire class can see it easily and where glare is minimal. It must be
kept clean between uses. You should write only on the upper two-
thirds of the board because students often have difficulty seeing
the bottom of the board over each other's heads. Printing or diagrams should be large enough to be seen from the back of the room,
and not too much information should be on the board at one time.
If the board is covered with information, chances are you are using
the wrong method and should switch to handouts or an overhead
projector. You should not waste time during class putting material
on the board that could have been prepared ahead of time on the
chalkboard, handouts, or transparencies.

Diagrams and pictures can be sketched on the chalkboard before class. Doing so not only saves time but permits you to draw a
neater sketch than might be produced under pressure and the eyes
of the students. If you wish to draw the picture while the students

are watching, you can at least put in some faint chalk lines before class to guide you during the actual drawing. Colored chalk helps make drawings more interesting and can be used to highlight important points. You need not apologize for lack of drawing skills; students don't expect instructors to be artists, and such apologies only draw attention to you rather than the subject matter.

Among the drawbacks of using the chalkboard are that it cannot be used with large groups and that the material usually cannot be saved until the next class. The fact that your back is to the students while writing on the board is a disadvantage because you lose contact with the class, and the class may have difficulty hearing what you are saying. Finally, this method is poor for the instructor who has poor handwriting, since the information may be lost because students cannot read what is written.

Overhead Transparencies

Transparencies are transparent sheets of acetate placed on an overhead projector that enlarges and projects the image onto a screen. Transparencies are easy to make, use, store, and transport and can be an asset to any teacher.

Transparencies can be used similarly to a chalkboard—for writing down spontaneous ideas, outlining class content, or doing math problems—but their use surpasses that of a chalkboard. Transparencies can be prepared beforehand to save class time and to help organize and illustrate content. Diagrams and drawings can be drawn or copied onto transparencies. Concepts can be illustrated. Lectures can be outlined. Charts and graphs can be presented. Cartoons can be projected for interest and illustration.

One of the features of the overhead projector is that it stands in front of the audience rather than within it, so that you can face the class while using it; thus, eye contact with students can be maintained. The room does not have to be dark, although it is often helpful to dim the lights around the screen. The projector is easy to use, requiring only manipulation of an on-off switch and a focus knob. Small portable projectors are available for teachers who go out on guest lectures and want to take their own audiovisual equipment.

It is easy to make your own transparencies if you keep a few points in mind. First, make sure you are using the right equipment. Some transparency sheets are designed to be used with marking pens; others are designed for thermofax machines or copying machines. If you try drawing on the wrong type of sheet, you may find that your ink bubbles up or disappears. If you try running the wrong type of sheet through a copying machine, the transparency may melt. If you are going to draw your own images, you have a choice of wax pencils like china markers, or colored ink pens. Ink is either nonpermanent (washable with water) or permanent (sometimes washable with alcohol). If you want to reuse the transparency sheet later for another purpose, be sure to use a pen with washable ink.

Whether you are drawing the image on the transparency or copying it from a printed page, keep the amount of information on the sheet to a minimum and make the image large enough that when it is projected students in the back of the room will be able to see it. A good rule of thumb is to make a picture or diagram fill the entire transparency sheet, with only one picture per sheet. If the transparency contains only words, each letter should be at least one fourth of an inch high, with no more than ten lines of printed material.

Avoid copying information from a printed book or magazine page or a typewritten sheet. Such pages present too much information for the students to take in, and the print is usually too small for them to see easily. If you want to type some information onto a transparency, type it on paper first, enlarge the type on a copier with an enlarging function, and then make a transparency.

Consult the audiovisual specialists or copy machine operators in your institution if you want to make a transparency on a copier. Making such copies usually requires loading the acetate sheets on top of the paper supply and then proceeding as you would to make any copy, but a little help or advice can keep you from breaking the machine or ruining your transparency.

Transparencies can also be made with overlays—additional acetate sheets that can be folded over the original to add new features or colors. A common use of overlays is with transparencies of anatomical figures. For example, the base sheet may show the gross anatomy of the heart chambers, and a hinged overlay placed on top of the original can show, with arrows, the direction of blood flow. Another overlay may indicate areas where various heart sounds originate.

Transparencies can be very creative, especially if you have artistic help. If you have produced a transparency worth saving for future classes, you may want to mount it in a cardboard frame that gives it some protection, enables you to handle it without touching the acetate, and reduces glare around the image.

Many commercially produced transparencies are available through media companies or textbook publishers. A number of basic textbooks have accompanying sets of transparencies that illustrate the main concepts of the book. Before purchasing large sets of transparencies, evaluate how much use will actually be made of them. If only a few in the set are really valuable, it might be more economical to make your own.

Just a few more tips about using the overhead projector: While you are showing a transparency, be careful that you are not blocking the students' view. You may be in the direct visual path of students sitting near the projector, so once you have turned the machine on, move around occasionally or move back close to the screen. If you have finished referring to one transparency and will not be using the next one for a while, remove the first one and turn the projector off. Doing so will conserve the light bulb and reduce distraction for the students. Finally, leave the transparency on screen long enough for students to read and absorb all the information. Nothing is quite as frustrating as having a transparency whisked away before one has had a chance to read or take notes on the material. If students don't trust you to leave the transparency on long enough, they will feverishly attempt to write down everything on the screen as fast as possible, at the expense of listening to what you have to say about it. You can control this behavior by covering up portions of the image until you get around to discussing them, or you can assure the students that you will not remove the transparency until they are ready.

At least one research study has demonstrated the value of using transparencies. Working with 104 engineering students in a geometry class, Chance (1961) divided the students into an experimental group taught by means of 200 transparencies and 800 overlays, and a control group taught by the usual instruction with the chalkboard (cited in Wendt & Butts, 1962). Chance found that the transparency group did significantly better than the chalkboard group and that the material was covered in less time with transparencies and with greater student attentiveness.

Slides

You may use slides to show pictures or to project diagrams, charts, and word concepts. Slides can be effective promoters of discussions, can help to make abstractions concrete, and can lend realism to an otherwise academic discussion. Occasionally you may want students to see a magazine picture or chart but hesitate to send them to the library just for that. Or perhaps you would like students to see certain illustrations in conjunction with the class presentation. In these cases, making slides of the material can be the answer. Any graphics that would help illustrate a lecture can be made into clear and colorful slides.

The advantages of slides over some other media are that they are inexpensive to make or buy, they are compact and easy to store, and they are easy to update and reorganize to fit changing class needs. The speed of slide presentation can be controlled by the teacher so that each frame can be discussed for the desired length of time. A remote-control extension allows you to walk around or stand in front of the class and still control the slides. It is also easy to back up to previous frames if a question arises pertaining to them. Slide projectors are lightweight and easy to carry.

The disadvantages of slides are that they can easily get dirty and smudged with fingerprints because they are so small, and they can get bent inside a malfunctioning projector. Projector bulbs don't last very long and are expensive to replace. Reduced room light is necessary to get a clear image on the screen, which makes it difficult for students to take notes. Also, the size of slide trays is not standardized, so a teacher's personal slide tray may not fit the projectors used in a particular institution. Thus, many teachers store slides in a box and then insert them in a tray before every use.

Before showing a set of slides to a class, you should carefully organize them to fit into the lecture, discussion, or module. The easiest way to organize a large group of slides is to place them on a tabletop slide previewer. This will enable you to see all the slides at once and select the order in which you want to show them. If you want to include some discussion time between slides but don't want to be bothered turning the projector off and on, you can obtain or make black slides that keep the screen clear yet block the projection light.

Use care to position the slides correctly in the tray, to avoid the surprise of upside down or sideways shots or backward lettering. It is often helpful to number the slides to keep them in order; the number itself can then be used as an indicator of how the slides should be positioned in the tray.

To prepare your own slides, you will probably need some advice or help from a media specialist in your institution. You may also consult books that explain the process step by step. In some institutions the production staff will actually make the slides for you if you write out what you want for a printed slide and provide the magazine pictures or charts that you want copied. Make sure that you obtain permission to use copyrighted materials, if necessary.

Prepared slides are also available from many sources, including media companies, medical and surgical supplies companies, and various public health organizations. Commercial slides are frequently offered in the form of slide-tapes. These narrated slide shows are more expensive but are often more useful in teaching many subjects because they depict nursing situations and lend themselves to the teaching of problem-solving and decision-making skills. They are also valuable for independent study.

Sound Filmstrips

Filmstrips are similar to slides in that they are still pictures on 35mm film, but instead of being physically separate pictures they are all connected on a strip in a sequential order that cannot be changed. The filmstrip projector advances each frame automatically or manually, and the accompanying audiotapes are synchronized for each frame. Although it is possible for teachers to produce their own filmstrips with a special camera, it is seldom done. Sound filmstrips can be purchased relatively inexpensively compared to films.

Audiotapes

Tape recorders and audiotapes can be used effectively to achieve a variety of educational purposes and have several advantages over other forms of technology. Although reel-to-reel tape recorders are still used to some extent in schools today, they are bulkier and more difficult to use than the smaller portable cassette recorders. Thus, the discussion of audiotapes in this section refers primarily to cassette tapes and recorders.

Tapes are valuable in helping students learn communication skills. Whether students are role playing a nurse-patient interaction or actually conversing with a real patient (taped with permission), a recording can capture the essence of the interaction, and the tape can be played back and analyzed for effective and ineffective communication patterns. A dramatization of a family interaction or of other case study material can be recorded for students to use as a basis for learning assessment and care planning.

You can record step-by-step skill instructions that students can use when they are alone during practice sessions; it is sometimes easier to listen to the tape while performing the skill rather than having to keep referring to a book. You can also tape speakers (with permission) and then play excerpts of the speeches in class. Sometimes excerpts of controversial information can spark lively class discussions.

A technique that some teachers find attractive is using a tape recorder to give students feedback on written assignments (Fredette, 1984). Rather than the impersonal feeling conveyed by comments written on a student's paper, the comments given in the instructor's voice carry an emphasis and intonation that will provide the student with needed reinforcement. Of course, this procedure requires that every student have access to a cassette recorder and supply the teacher with a blank tape.

Students can make good use of audiotapes by taping lectures or other class proceedings so that they can concentrate on what is being said and done rather than on note taking. Some instructors feel uncomfortable with tape recorders running during class, but when students are freed from note taking the classroom becomes a livelier place with more give and take. Teachers may also benefit from making their own tapes of classes for self-evaluation.

Audiotapes can play a large part in independent study programs. The students can listen to tapes or can watch slides or filmstrips with synchronized tapes and learn at their own pace. They can rewind or fast-forward the tapes as desired to meet their needs.

Other advantages of audiotapes and cassette recorders are that they are small and easy to carry and store, they are easy to use, they are relatively inexpensive, and they can usually be run by either battery or electricity.

Among the disadvantages of cassette tapes is the fact that the sound quality of many units is not too good, especially for recording music. The tape itself can sometimes become unwound and tangled inside the recorder, necessitating splicing and repair that in many cases ruins the message. And most important, listening to a tape without any visual effects can be soporific unless the topic is lively or the speaker witty.

One study that attests to the educational value of audiotapes was conducted by Rowsey and Mason in 1975. They researched the relative learning of two groups of college biology students: those taught by means of conventional lectures and labs, and those taught by audiotape lectures and individual exercises with instructions also given via audiotape. The researchers found that the audio-tutorial group had significantly higher scores both on immediate achievement tests and on retention tests given 11 weeks later.

Videotapes

Most educational institutions today have videocassette recorders (VCRs) that are used for playing commercially prepared videocassettes. In addition, many schools and hospitals have the cameras and recording equipment needed to make their own videotapes.

Videotapes are becoming more popular and are replacing films in many cases, probably because they are less expensive, less fragile, and easier to use and store than 16mm films. Videotapes have many educational applications, and videotape technology can be used in many creative ways.

Well-known speakers or guest lecturers can be taped (with their permission) and the lecture played for other groups or for future classes on the same subject. Demonstrations of skills and procedures by in-house faculty or guests can be recorded and saved. It is much easier for a large group to see a skill on a videotape shown above their heads than to see the details of a live demonstration in front of the room. If the demonstration is to be shown to several groups, a videotape also ensures that the procedure is done exactly the same each time so that each group receives the same instruction.

If the hospital or hospitals that your school is affiliated with have videotaping equipment, you may be able to borrow it (and the hospital's technical assistance) to make tapes of areas of the hospital that are relatively inaccessible to learners, such as the emergency department, operating room, or intensive care unit. Orientation tapes or tapes that actually record the performance of patient care (with permission from the people being filmed) can be made. For example, you may go into an empty operating room suite and make a videotape to show scrubbing and gowning procedures as well as the setup of the room.

If you film in another hospital or agency, you should make sure that the filming equipment is compatible with the viewing equipment in your institution. For example, if you film on 3/4-inch cassette equipment when your school has 1/2-inch cassette hard-

ware, you will have a problem unless the technical staff can copy
the tape onto 1/2-inch cassettes.

Within the educational institution, videotaping can also be
used creatively. Students can be filmed during role-playing exercises while learning such things as communication skills. Smith,
Margolius, and Ross (1982) described the making and testing of a
package of videotapes on therapeutic communication. The faculty
prepared a tape consisting of six vignettes depicting nurse-patient
interactions, both therapeutic and nontherapeutic. They researched
the effectiveness of this tape in helping students learn and apply
communication theory by having the students take a multiple-
choice test before and after viewing the tape and also having the
students role play a nurse-patient interaction before and after seeing the videotape. These role-playing tests were also videotaped
for grading purposes. The researchers discovered that the videotape with the six vignettes had a significant positive effect on the
acquisition of communication theory and its application in simulated clinical settings.

Simulation tapes can be made to help prepare students for
clinical experiences. For example, Shaffer and Pfeiffer (1980) prepared videotapes of simulations in community health nursing.
Any number of simulated patient situations could be filmed in a
college nursing laboratory and used as introductions to commonly
occurring clinical situations. These tapes could be shown in a class
setting or prepared for individual student use.

Evaluation of student learning is also an appropriate domain
for videotaping. Richards et al (1981) used videotapes of simulated
psychiatric nursing scenarios to measure students' abilities to diagnose problems, list interventions, and chart appropriate nurse's
notes. Eggert (1975) and Rogers (1976) both used videotapes to
evaluate interpersonal skills. The advantage to using tapes for
evaluating clinical skills is that the testing situations can be controlled and the variables, especially those that produce undue
student anxiety, can be reduced. The major disadvantage is that
videotaping students may initially make them anxious and preoc-
cupied with the image they are projecting (Finley, 1979; Memmer,
1979). This self-consciousness makes students less likely to perform at their highest level of ability. Sufficient practice sessions
should be offered to enable students to get accustomed to the
taping process so that they can ignore that aspect and concentrate
on the behaviors being evaluated.

As with audiotaping, videotaping has a role to play in faculty self-evaluation. For student-teachers and teachers at any point in their careers, seeing a videotape of a class they have just taught can be an eye-opening and valuable experience, especially if a master teacher is on hand to help evaluate the taped performance and give suggestions.

Videotaping has several advantages over other media. On a videotape the teacher can still maintain eye contact with the class and provide something of a personal touch, even though the performance is not live. Also, motion enhances the realism of the situation and often increases interest.

All students watching a videotape are exposed to the same teaching, even though the students may be in different class sections at different times. This reduces the problem of slightly different information and emphasis being given for different class sections taking the same examinations.

Once a lecture or dramatization is captured on videotape, it can be used for independent study as well as classroom teaching and can be used at the students' own pace. They can replay and freeze frames according to their needs. In classroom settings, the teacher may choose to freeze the action and discuss what has just been played before proceeding. Although videotaping hardware can be costly, the software is relatively inexpensive, and cassettes are reusable.

The disadvantages of videotapes include the fact that communication is only one-way and students cannot interact with the media; they become passive recipients of information. This effect can be minimized by instructor involvement before, during, or after showing the videotape. In comparison with live lectures, lectures on videotape have a set pace that may be inappropriate for a particular group of students. A live lecturer can change pace to meet the perceived needs of the audience; a taped lecturer cannot.

In addition to the high cost of equipment, the costs of maintenance are high. Further costs are involved if technicians are required for producing tapes. Faculty may prepare subject matter and scripts for the taping, but usually the media team in the institution gets involved in taping procedures. However, an institution may decide to use only commercially prepared videotapes and therefore only have to pay for the tapes, the VCR, and the monitor, bypassing the expenses of equipment needed to make in-house tapes.

Some research has been done to test the effectiveness of videotapes in learning. In 1973 Siegel presented a psychology lesson to college students using four groups and four methods: lecture, printed notes, videotape, and audiotape. He found that the group who learned from printed notes performed best on the examination, followed by the lecture and videotape groups and last by the audiotape group. A retention test given 2 months later placed the groups in the same order.

VanMondfrans et al (1972) developed a series of 15 videotaped lectures and demonstrations for an introductory nursing course. They taught a control group with live lectures and demonstrations and an experimental group with the videotapes. Test results showed that for much of the material, videotapes were more effective than live lectures in meeting the objectives, particularly when skill demonstrations were involved. Both methods were found to be acceptable to the students.

Another nurse researcher investigated the performance of two groups of nursing students who were learning to use the Denver Developmental Screening Test (Koniak, 1985). The control group was taught via lecture/demonstration, while the experimental group was taught via the autotutorial approach with considerable content given by videotape. Students in the autotutorial group scored significantly higher on the performance test than the students taught by traditional methods.

Films

Films used to be considered the most sophisticated of the audiovisuals, capable of accomplishing many different learning objectives. Although they are still valuable, they are rivalled today by videotapes and interactive video-computer programs.

Films can be used to enhance learning in a number of ways. They can help demonstrate complex skills and behaviors more realistically than many other media and can demonstrate desired behaviors in a real-life context. Theoretical content can be applied on the screen, thus enhancing retention and transfer of learning. Motion pictures can actually show the problem solving process, not only visually, but with a commentary on people's thoughts and motives. Films not only show action but also demonstrate cause and effect and the history behind actions. Because films can move into the future to show results of present actions, they can be used to shape student attitudes, an important part of socialization into a profession.

Films are useful in showing events over time; they can depict the course of a lengthy illness or condense a person's entire life into 1 hour. They also show relationships between things that have been learned in isolation and help bring material into a unified whole. They reinforce what has been learned and extend the material beyond the bare bones of what has been learned in theory. Motion pictures may be good economic substitutes for field trips and can be used for individual as well as group learning.

Research has revealed that class time can be saved by teaching with films; for example, students can learn the same concepts faster by means of film than they can by lecture (Wendt & Butts, 1962). Small and large groups can benefit equally well from motion pictures, and the attention of the students is easily held. Probably the greatest advantage of films is that they can convey almost any type of learning, whether learning of concepts, rules, facts, procedures, visual identifications, or attitudes and opinions (Allen, 1967).

A major disadvantage of films is that students are again thrust into a passive role of watching but not interacting. The teacher is limited to making comments before or after the film because it cannot effectively be interrupted. If the teacher makes comments about specific segments of the film after it is over, the students may not have a clear recollection of the portion of the film being discussed. Students are limited in their ability to take notes during the film because the room has to be dark.

Both projection equipment and films are expensive to purchase or rent, and maintenance costs are also high. Even previewing of films is a costly process today. Faculty may not be familiar with how to run a projector, so technical staff may have to be involved. If teachers who know little about film projection are forced to be responsible for the procedure, they may not know what to do if problems crop up, such as film jumping out of the sprockets or fuzzy sound, and they may unwittingly do damage to the equipment. Projection equipment is heavy and not really very portable unless it is on a cart.

Finally, some films run for an hour or more, which means that they are too long for some class periods. An instructor should check the running time before ordering a film. Films should be purchased with caution in light of the expense. Many films, especially in the health field, are quickly outdated and will sit on the shelf after 2 or 3 years. Rentals may be the better option for material that could soon date itself.

The relative effectiveness of films as a teaching strategy has received attention by a considerable number of researchers. In 1956

Greenhill and McNiven (cited in Wendt & Butts, 1962) conducted one of the few studies that explored the use of a medium without comparing it to another teaching method. They studied the perceived usefulness of films shown to 473 high school seniors. They discovered that the more a viewer can picture himself or herself using the content of the film, the more he or she will learn from the material. This finding speaks to the importance of helping students understand, even before seeing a film, how they will be able to use the information.

Several studies that compared films to traditional teaching methods found no significant differences in learning outcomes (Anderson & Montgomery, 1959 and Drury, 1959 cited in Wendt & Butts, 1962; Huckabay, Cooper & Neal, 1977; Schorow, Osborne & Kelsey, 1971). Popham and Sadnavitch in 1961 (cited in Wendt & Butts, 1962) reported that high school physics students who were taught by traditional methods performed significantly better than peers taught with films.

Yock and Erlandson (1957) compared the effectiveness of film and demonstrations in dental classes. They taught a particular skill by three means: film alone, demonstration alone, and a combination of film and demonstration. Not surprisingly, the combination group fared significantly better at the end of the unit. Although neither method proved superior, it was demonstrated that they can be used together successfully.

Summary of Research

A lot of research has been done over the last 30 years or so in an attempt to compare teaching by means of audiovisuals to so-called conventional teaching, which usually consists of lecture or lecture/discussion. In 1976 Watts studied the effect of lectures versus audiovisual presentation versus independent study on learning outcomes in a college sexuality course. The results showed that the lecture group learned significantly better than the other two groups.

Jensen and Knauff (1977) used geometry students to research the effectiveness of a multimedia approach (cited in Roberts & Thurston, 1984; 22). They found that the multimedia approach was particularly effective for presenting complex as opposed to simpler material.

A college course in descriptive geometry was the setting for a 1979 study by Rankowski and Galey, who tested the effects of the lecture versus multimedia approach. The results showed higher mean scores for students in the multimedia group.

Thompson studied nursing students in 1972. One group received content by means of lectures, while another group was taught with a multimedia autotutorial approach that included films, videotapes, slide-tape programs, and programmed booklets. One year later, the investigator found no significant difference in retention of the learned material.

Another group of nursing students was studied by Roberts and Thurston (1984). Material on nursing care for spinal cord injuries was presented in two modes: (1) lecture and (2) lecture plus overhead transparencies, slides, diagrams, drawings, and models. The researchers reported no significant differences in initial learning, but the experimental group (lecture plus multimedia) retained significantly more information 3 weeks later. There is some evidence, then, in favor of the worth of multimedia presentations in the classroom.

Unfortunately, the research findings do not present a clear picture of the effectiveness of audiovisual learning. The evidence conflicts, with audiovisuals found to be more effective than traditional methods in some studies and less effective in others. There are several explanations of this paradoxical picture. The first consideration in evaluating a research report is "What is being taught?" It seems evident that the effectiveness of a teaching method will vary with the content, and several studies bear out this conclusion. It may be that some of the technologies are effective in teaching complex information but not effective in teaching simple facts and concepts or that audiovisual media may be especially suited to teaching skills rather than logical thought processes. Further research into the relative effectiveness of the various audiovisual media in enhancing various kinds of learning is needed.

Lack of definition and description of the control group in existing studies also causes confusion. The control groups are often described as receiving "traditional" teaching methods. This term usually refers (on the college level) to lecture/discussions with use of the chalkboard and printed materials. But this may not always be the case, and it is important to know the exact nature of the "traditional" method in evaluating the research findings.

It is also important to know, yet it is seldom mentioned, just how similar or different the methods are that are being compared. For example, a study may compare lectures to videotapes in effects on learning, but what is the nature of the videotapes? Are they tapes of the same person giving the same lecture being given live to the control group? Are the videotapes commercially prepared and therefore perhaps do not cover all the same material as the lecture? Do the videotapes present the subject in an innovative manner vastly different from the lecture? Perhaps what the researcher is actually studying is not just the medium but the approach to learning; if this is the case, the research consumer should be aware of it.

Another concern in evaluating and interpreting the research on audiovisuals is lack of clarity about the criteria against which learning is being measured. If the criterion test is measuring only knowledge of facts and understanding of concepts, it may not be surprising to find no significant differences between teaching methods. Maybe if different criteria were used and different tests were given, such as tests of understanding, problem solving, or logical thinking, it would become clearer as to which methods best produce which type of learning. Further testing of these areas is needed.

We can conclude that no single audiovisual medium is effective for all teaching purposes (Gagné, 1970). Instructors can be guided somewhat by research carried out in circumstances similar to those in which they will be teaching, and they can rely on their knowledge of educational objectives to tell them which methods will achieve their aims.

Teacher Responsibilities

Whether showing slides, videotapes, filmstrips, or films, you must preview the software to ensure that it helps meet course objectives. You may find that you only need or want to show a part of the program and can skip the rest without sacrificing any valuable information. Arrangements to show the software in class must be made ahead of time to ensure getting a projector or other equipment when it is needed. You should prepare the class adequately before showing the software. They should be told about the purpose of the program, special points to look for, and knowledge they can expect to gain from it. You should try to tie in the audiovisual to previous content covered and should point out material that should already be familiar to the students.

It is a good idea to stay in the room while software is being shown, even if a technician is running the equipment. Your presence communicates that you think the program is worthwhile, that it holds your interest, and that it is not just being used to allow you time off from the classroom. While you are in the room, you can also be alert to student reactions and may perceive that certain segments need to be explained when the showing is over.

Media programs should always be discussed afterward. Try to avoid programs that fill the whole class period and allow no time for discussion. Discussion and reaction after the showing can provide valuable reinforcement of the learning. If that discussion must take place the day after the audiovisual is shown, it loses some of its interest and purpose.

Audiovisuals are a boon to education. When used in conjunction with other teaching strategies, they add interest and quality to a class. The teacher, however, always retains responsibility for the proper preparation and use of materials so that they enhance rather than detract from the learning process.

References

Allen WH: Media stimulus and types of learning. *Audiovisual Instruction* 1967; 12:27–31.

Eggert LL: Challenge exams in interpersonal skills. *Nurs Outlook* 1975; 23:707–710.

Finley B, Kim KK, Mynatt S: Maximizing videotaped learning of interpersonal skills. *J Nurs Educ* (Jan) 1979; 18:33–41.

Fredette SL: Individualized clinical teaching via the tape recorder. *Image* 1984; 16:80–83.

Gagné RM: *The Conditions of Learning.* Holt, Rinehart and Winston, 1970.

Huckabay L, Cooper P, Neal M: Effect of specific teaching techniques. *Nurs Res* 1977; 28:380–385.

Jamison D, Suppes P, Wells S: The effectiveness of alternative instructional media: a survey. *Rev Educ Res* (Winter) 1974; 44:1–67.

Koniak D: Autotutorial and lecture-demonstration instruction: a comparative analysis of the effects upon students' learning of a developmental assessment skill. *West J Nurs Res* 1985; 7:80–100.

MacManaway LA: Using lecture scripts. *Universities Quarterly* 1968; 22:327–336.

Memmer MK: Television replay: a tool for students to learn to evaluate their own proficiency in using sterile technique. *J Nurs Educ* (Oct) 1979; 18:35–42.

Rankowski CA, Galey M: Effectiveness of multimedia in teaching descriptive geometry. *ECTJ* 1979; 27:114–120.

Richards A et al: Videotape as an evaluation tool. *Nurs Outlook* 1981; 29:35–38.

Roberts K, Thurston H: Teaching methodologies: knowledge acquisition and retention. *J Nurs Educ* (Jan) 1984; 23:21–26.

Rogers S: Testing the RN student's skills. *Nurs Outlook* 1976; 24:446–449.

Rowsey RE, Mason WH: Immediate achievement and retention in audio-tutorial versus conventional lecture-laboratory instruction. *J Res Science Teaching* 1975; 12:393–397.

Schorow M, Osborne J, Kelsey H: Training nurses for coronary care practice. *Nurs Outlook* 1971; 19:95–97.

Shaffer MK, Pfeiffer IL: You too can prepare videotapes for instruction. *J Nurs Educ* (March) 1980; 19:23–27.

Siegel HB: McLuhan, mass media, and education. *J Exper Educ* 1973; 41:68–70.

Smith IK, Margolius F, Ross GR: Development and validation of a trigger tape on therapeutic communication. *J Nurs Educ* (April) 1982; 21:42–47.

Thompson M: Learning: A comparison of traditional and autotutorial methods. *Nurs Res* 1972; 21:453–457.

Van Mondfrans AP, Sorenson C, Reed CL: Live or taped? *Nurs Outlook* 1972; 20:652–653.

Watts PR: Comparison of three human sexuality teaching methods used in university health classes. *Res Quarterly* 1976; 48:187–190.

Wendt PR, Butts GK: Audiovisual materials. *Rev Educ Res* 1962; 32:141–151.

Yock DH, Erlandson FL: The effectiveness of visual aids in dental teaching. *J Educ Res* 1958; 52:11–15.

Chapter 11

Computer Technology

Computer use in nursing education is increasing greatly as hardware costs decrease and software proliferates. Some colleges and universities have mainframe computers—large computers with tremendous memory capacity costing hundreds of thousands of dollars—but probably more institutions are investing in microcomputers, which cost a few thousand dollars and are eminently suitable for student use. Nursing departments in many schools are allocating capital funds or obtaining grant money to buy microcomputers and software for student use.

Although the investment is large, the return in student learning can be great, and educators are still finding new ways of using computers that will certainly offset the investment. More and more students graduating from high school have been exposed to computers or are computer literate; now it is time for nursing faculty to learn about computers and how they can be used to enhance teaching.

Computer systems used in nursing programs include large mainframe systems such as PLATO, based at the University of Illinois, a project of Control Data Corporation (Jenkins & Dankert, 1981; Mahr & Kadner, 1984). PLATO (Programmed Logic for Automated Teaching Operations) is a time-sharing computer dedicated to educational purposes. PLATO terminals are in many schools in the United States and Canada. Students at distant geographical locations can log into the mainframe computer and call up various programs used in their curriculum.

The individual microcomputers that many nursing programs are purchasing have several advantages over the large mainframe systems. They can be bought a few at a time as money is allocated, and if something goes wrong, only one computer is out of commission as opposed to complete shutdown of all terminals in a mainframe system. A great deal of educational software for nursing students is currently being written for microcomputers.

A microcomputer consists of a central processing unit (CPU) where the "intellectual" and some memory functions take place. Programs (educational lessons, for example) are loaded into the CPU from a disk where they are stored. Output from the CPU can also be stored on disks, if desired. For instance, a student may be asked to view a program that contains a case study and simulation. The student inserts the program disk, which contains all the educational information, into a disk drive that relays the information to the CPU. The CPU sends information to the monitor, where the student can read the messages. To move the program along, or to answer questions asked by the program, the student presses keys on the keyboard. If the program permits student answers to be saved and recorded, they are saved on a separate disk.

Besides the hardware already mentioned, the system may include a printer. If students are using a word-processing package to prepare a paper or nursing care plan, they need a printer to obtain a permanent (hard) copy of the manuscript.

Educational Uses

Computers have many educational uses and applications. They can teach at any level of learning, from knowledge and comprehension up through application, analysis, and synthesis. They can be programmed to teach problem solving and decision making.

One of the biggest advantages of computers over most of the other audiovisual technologies is that the student is an active participant in the learning process, able to manipulate information, take action in vicarious situations, and use trial and error. The active participant role enhances learning and retention (see Chapter 2).

In addition to their teaching role, computers can be used to monitor student progress, evaluate student responses, and tailor student remedial work. The teacher can obtain a record of the kinds of responses that students make to questions in the computer program and can see the paths into which the students' thinking is taking them. Errors in reasoning or calculations can be identified so that appropriate help can be given to the student.

The primary computer application for students in a nursing program is *computer-assisted instruction*, or learning by means of computer programs. *Computer-managed instruction* is also important in education; in this mode the computer is primarily used by the instructor to organize and keep records of student learning. Finally, learning to use the computer as a tool is an important general aspect of the students' education, as the knowledge will have many future applications. Graduates of nursing programs will be expected to learn how to use computers in providing patient care, and they must obtain the necessary basic computer education in college so that they can apply their learning in the workplace.

Let us look at each of these three aspects of computer use (computer-assisted instruction, computer-managed instruction, and using the computer as a tool) in greater detail.

Computer-Assisted Instruction

Computer-assisted instruction, also known as CAI, occurs in several formats, or modes. The simplest level is the *drill and practice* mode. In this format, students have already learned certain information, either through computer programs or other teaching methods, and are now presented with repetition and application of the information. This mode particularly lends itself to teaching mathematical calculations. The students may have received a lecture/demonstration on solving math problems in pharmacology. They are then sent to the computer, which presents problem after problem to be solved. The computer program tells the student whether the answers are correct and may go so far as to diagnose the problem if the answers are incorrect. Drill and practice can also be used in learning drug names and actions, in learning medical terminology, or in any situation requiring memorization of facts and concepts (Lorenz, 1983). It is probably the mode in which the least amount of software has been written, because of the low level of learning that it represents.

The second mode in which educational computer software may be written is the *tutorial* mode. The program "tutors" or teaches the student a body of knowledge by presenting information and asking questions, giving hints if the student gets stuck. Tutorials are most useful in teaching material at the rule and concept level. Tutorial software can free faculty members from teaching some of the routine basic material, which becomes tedious after lecturing on it the first few times, and allows them to use their time more creatively and productively on higher-level learning. At the same time, students may find that tutorials on basic information are more interesting and fun than an instructor's lectures.

Any information taught by means of lecture could potentially be written as a computer tutorial program. That does not mean that all basic classroom lectures should be turned into computer instruction, but it is possible to do so.

A segment of a tutorial program on immobility may appear something like this:

Computer: As described, immobility takes its toll on almost every body system, and nurses must use preventive measures to protect the patient from those effects. Let's review some of the material covered.

              If the nurse encourages a patient to force fluids, which hazards of immobility is he/she trying to prevent?

Student: (kidney stones, or renal calculi, and urinary infection)

Computer: Right! A high flow rate through the urinary system helps to prevent renal calculi and urinary infection.

              Which particular fluid would be most effective in helping to prevent urinary infection?

Student: (cranberry juice or prune juice)

Computer: Good! Juices that help produce an acidic urine reduce the chances of urinary infection in an immobile patient . . .

Tutorials thus take the form of an interactive lecture with built-in feedback and can be developed very creatively, especially if graphics are used.

Software can also be written in *game* mode. Just as board games, card games, and trivia games can be used to teach nursing, so can computer games. Relatively few nursing game programs have been written, probably because good games are not easy to devise and because software specialists have been concentrating their efforts on other modes.

The *simulation and problem-solving* mode is one of the most exciting and available forms of computer software. Simulations of real-world experiences provide students with the opportunity to learn how to solve clinical problems and make sound decisions. Computer simulations can provide students with all the details about a particular patient situation and then ask them to assess the patient, arrive at diagnoses, plan interventions, and evaluate care.

Simulations can demand decisions in emergency situations and can show the results of good or poor decisions.

The advantage of providing these learning experiences via computer is that students can all be exposed to the same learning situation, which is not the case in a clinical setting. Even more important, students can take risks and make mistakes with no danger to the patient. In a computer simulation the student is functioning in a controlled world where unexpected variables and pressures characteristic of the clinical area do not occur. Of course, the disadvantage of computer simulations is that instructors find out only what students might do or are capable of doing in a situation, not how they would actually perform in reality.

A computer simulation might be formatted in the following way:

Description of patient situation.

Student selects (from a list) which data should be collected.

Computer provides feedback about the choices selected.

Student uses the correct data to arrive at a nursing diagnosis (selected from a list).

Computer provides feedback on selection.

Student selects (from a list) nursing goals appropriate to the situation.

Computer responds to each selection as to why it would or wouldn't be a realistic goal.

Student selects (from a list) nursing actions that would help solve the patient's problems.

Computer responds with the positive and negative effects of each action on the patient.

Student selects (from a list) evaluation criteria that indicate success of nursing actions.

Computer provides feedback on criteria.

This is a simplified format of a computer simulation using the nursing process. Actual programs are much more complex and allow for branching or relooping, meaning that whenever students lose their grasp of the situation they can move back to an earlier part of the program to brush up on information or retrace their actions. They may be able to branch into a tutorial mode for reinforcement of background material, or they may be automatically moved into alternate paths depending on the patterns of their responses (Mahr, 1984; Reynolds, 1984).

Many other kinds of simulations exist besides this type of case study/nursing process format. A simulation may consist of a cardiac arrest scenario, with the student having to take emergency action, or it could be a simulated interaction with a psychiatric patient. The possibilities are almost limitless.

Finally, computer programs can be written in the *examination* mode. Questions, with or without situations, can be written in multiple-choice, true/false, or fill-in-the-blank format. Rationales can be given following the answers, if desired. This type of examination can be used for practice purposes, especially practice for state board examinations. Such quizzes provide students with instant feedback on their performance. There are also programs that teachers can use to construct tests used for grading purposes. Students take the test on the computer, which compiles the answers for all students and does an item analysis and statistical breakdown. This function of the computer leads us into the second aspect of computer use: computer-managed instruction.

Computer-Managed Instruction

Teachers can use computers to manage, prepare, and organize educational experiences. Examinations like the ones just mentioned can fall under the heading of computer-managed instruction. Any system of record keeping can be included in this category as well, such as calculating and recording grades, ordering class ranks, and recording student profiles. Nursing faculty may use computers to schedule clinical agencies and assignments, assign rotation through clinical experiences, and even record anecdotal records of student experiences. Although computer management of instruction has been done mostly in the administrative offices of schools of nursing up until now, more of it will be done by teachers in their own offices or homes as microcomputer use expands among nursing faculty.

The use of *authoring systems* will also expand the use of computers among nursing instructors. Writing computer programs used to be exclusively the domain of people with a good background in computer languages such as BASIC, PASCAL, COBOL, and FORTRAN. Now teachers without programming skills can develop

CAI through authoring packages. Programmers lay the ground-work for a particular CAI package, and faculty need only insert their material into the program and learn some simple commands to individualize it for their purposes.

NEMAS (Nursing Education Module Authoring System), put out by Lippincott Co., and Microinstructor, by Mosbysystems, are examples of authoring systems. They allow instructors to develop simulation software in their specialty by inserting content as indi-cated by the authoring manual. Although an authoring system may be expensive, a plethora of software can be developed from it, thus justifying the expense.

It is not advisable for teachers without programming expertise or access to an authoring system to try to develop their own soft-ware for student use. The software so produced often appears amateurish and may have many built-in problems. Also, it takes about 300 hours of programming (without an authoring system) to create 1 hour of CAI (Brose, 1984), which makes it very expensive—often more expensive than commercially produced software.

Using the Computer as a Tool

Today's students will probably at some time in their nursing ca-reers use computers as part of a hospital information system. Hos-pitals are using mainframe computers as well as microcomputers to keep records for data bases. Nurses using such systems will have to learn how to enter physicians' orders and to order lab tests, diets, and drugs. They will be required to send messages to other depart-ments and other nursing units, and they will have to learn how to chart medications and nursing care as well as formulate nursing care plans (Edmunds, 1985). Many hospitals have computer termi-nals at the nurses' stations, where all these data are loaded in and accessed. In the future, nurses may carry pocket-sized computers on which they can enter data right at the patient's bedside.

Nurses can enter data into hospital information systems by two basic means. One is typing in the information on the keyboard, which is obviously time consuming. The other method is using a light pen. After an access code name or number and the patient's name are typed into the computer, a menu, or list of topics, ap-pears. For example, the list may look like this:

update physician's orders

enter lab tests

chart drugs

update nursing care plan

update nurse's notes

change diet

All of the possibilities for entering or retrieving data may appear on the menu. The nurse simply runs the light pen across the desired line. If the line is "update physician's orders," the screen will change and indicate how one is to enter the new orders. A hard copy of all current orders can then be printed out on the nearby printer if desired.

The best way to prepare students to use the computer as a professional tool is to teach it to them in a hospital that has a computerized information system. However, many clinical facilities where teaching is done do not yet have computers at the nurses' stations. The next best approach is to introduce students to computers by means of CAI so that they become familiar with general computer commands, with menu-driven programs, and with types of information that computers can handle. Thiele and Baldwin (1985) describe a CAI simulation that familiarizes students with hospital information systems. The use of such systems can also be discussed in various nursing courses.

No matter how much students are taught about computer use in hospitals, they will still have to be oriented to the particular computer and computer programs used in the hospitals or agencies in which they will be employed; that is the function of the hospital's staff development department.

The responsibility of the nursing faculty is to help students understand general computer functions and applications to nursing and to help them learn the content and process of nursing through CAI. Students do not all have to become computer literate to the point of being able to write computer programs.

Advantages of Computer Instruction

The primary advantage of computers is that they allow the student to interact in the learning situation; he or she can respond to questions, manipulate variables, or select appropriate items from a menu, all of which provide activity for the student and make learning more interesting, memorable, and valuable.

Computers can also individualize learning to an extraordinary degree. Not only does the student usually work alone at the computer and have the freedom to use whichever programs are available at the preferred rate of speed, but he or she also can receive individual help by means of branching within the programs. In a well-written program, if a student is already familiar with a certain portion of the material, he or she can skip ahead or move into a more advanced side track. On the other hand, if a student is having difficulty, branching may permit him or her to review certain segments of the program or branch into a tutorial lesson. Individual learning needs can truly be met if a variety of high-quality software is available.

Computer-assisted instruction can also enhance a student's self-esteem in several ways. First, the student is in control of the computer, especially in relation to the pace of learning. Between the controlled pace and the step-by-step increments of learning (as in programmed instruction), the student is quite likely to be successful, a phenomenon that is rare for some students.

The feedback from computer programs can also be rewarding. The computer can reply to the student's answers with statements like "Good job, Judy!" or "Tom, you have really learned that well" or "You're right!" Such instant positive feedback is not always given by teachers, but the computer never forgets to reward the student, if it is so programmed. Wrong answers trigger nonpunitive feedback. The computer screen may say, "Sorry, that's incorrect; try again, Robin" or "You need a little more review of this material before proceeding." The immediate feedback, whether positive or negative, is invaluable. The use of the student's name gives the impression of a human teacher providing the feedback, and many people, even educators, enjoy seeing the computer use their name once in a while.

The nonjudgmental nature and endless patience of the computer are also important advantages. If the student takes four tries to get the right answer, the computer will still never make him or her feel worthless or stupid. Assuming that other students are not watching, the student's peers need never know that he or she had difficulty with the material. Students thus become less afraid of making mistakes and less embarrassed about taking more time to learn the material.

Records of students' performances on simulations or practice tests can be kept on the computer. The teacher can keep track of the ease or difficulty with which students are moving through the programs and then provide individual counseling where needed or spend more instructional time on an area that is perplexing many students.

Computers can also be available to students for more hours than the instructor is. A computer lab in a school of nursing may still be open at 10 P.M. when teachers are at home. This flexibility of computer learning time may make educational experiences more available to students who have part-time jobs or family responsibilities.

It is also possible for larger numbers of students to be taught with the same-size faculty. To put it another way, faculty time can be saved and the educational process can be less costly. These factors may not be priorities in all schools, but the trend in nursing education, as in other fields, is certainly toward cost containment and increasing efficiency in teaching. Even if saving of faculty time is not stressed from an economic standpoint, it may be important from a scholarly viewpoint. If faculty are freed from some routine lectures, they will have more time for research and contributions to the science of nursing. Also, if a faculty is subject to frequent turnover of instructors, computer programs can help to provide curricular stability.

Disadvantages of Computer Instruction

There are disadvantages to CAI, although some of them are being overcome as more is learned about computer use and as more nurse educators become computer experts. The initial and sometimes overwhelming disadvantage is cost. Unless a school can afford large capital outlays or can secure grant monies, the large-scale purchase of computers may be impossible. Even if hardware is affordable, the costs of software can be prohibitive.

Good-quality software usually costs hundreds of dollars, and for that price only a few disks may be provided. Some companies give permission to make unlimited copies of disks; others make copy-protected disks that prevent people from making free copies. Inexpensive software is often available from other schools or individuals, and program exchanges may be possible, but in these cases the software is sometimes of poor quality and often provides the same type of learning that could be obtained from a programmed instruction book. Such software does not usually have any graphics and may have minimal branching (Zeimer, 1984).

Another problem with both hardware and software is lack of compatibility and transferability between companies. A school with an investment in one company's hardware may find that it cannot use some desirable software from another company, or the school that has microcomputers may be attracted to programs written for a mainframe computer. Rapid change in hardware and software may be a problem in itself. Microcomputers purchased today may be almost obsolete in 5 years. A program bought today because it is the only one available on a certain subject may be replaced by much superior software in a year or two, when it may be difficult to justify the purchase of more software on the same subject. The limited choice of high-quality software is a problem at present, but at the rate that nurses are becoming computer literate and collaborating with expert programmers, this should become less of a problem in the future.

Computer use also has some disadvantages from a student's standpoint. Many schools have a few microcomputers but not enough for the number of students in the program. Therefore, users have to wait their turn to get at a computer, and the computers may not be available when the students have the free time to use them. Schools of nursing have an obligation to purchase more computers, increase the hours of their availability, or decrease the students' computer assignments.

The fact that computer assignments usually require on-campus time can be a drawback, especially for commuter schools. Textbooks and programmed instruction can be taken home and studied, but many students do not have computers at home—or at least computers that are compatible with those of the school of nursing. Students may not be allowed to take the school's program disks home with them. Again, this whole situation may change in the future with more students owning computers and software becoming available for take-home work.

The time it takes for a student to use an educational program may also be a drawback in some situations. An average student using a program as it was designed to be used may learn the material in less time than it would take to learn it in a traditional classroom. But sometimes the time variable backfires. Students may stop to take notes on the computer tutorials (Van Dongen & Van Dongen, 1984), and lack of typing skill may slow some students down on programs that require a lot of answers to be keyboarded. However, if CAI is being used appropriately, as an adjunct to and not a substitute for all other methods of instruction, extensive note taking from computer programs should be unnecessary.

Evaluating Computer Software

With large numbers of software packages now coming on the market, many of them of questionable quality, the educator must be able to intelligently evaluate what each program has to offer and whether it will meet curricular objectives. It is helpful, as Smith (1985) suggests, to look at each program from the perspective of not only the instructor but also both strong and weak students.

The first criterion that any computer program must meet is factual accuracy. The instructor should go through the entire program checking for accuracy and currency of content. The teacher should also evaluate the "fit" between the material and the course objectives.

Second, the instructor should pay attention to the clarity with which the content is presented. Both the lesson material and the commands should be clear. Programs that are easy to use, especially menu-driven programs that give step-by-step instructions on the screen, are termed "user friendly." Students should be able to go through a program with no outside help once they have had an initial orientation.

A program is usually accompanied by a manual or user's guide. This documentation also should be clearly written, have an easy-to-use index, and contain a problem-solving section for students who run into problems. From the teacher's perspective, the manual should include information about the type and level of student for whom the program is designed, objectives of the lesson material, and an estimate of the average amount of time it should take students to complete the program. The manual should explain whether copies of the disks can be legally made, what arrangements exist for replacement of damaged disks, and what peripherals (such as a second disk drive or printer) are necessary.

The second time a teacher goes through the program, he or she should evaluate it from a student's perspective. Is the program interesting and maybe even fun? Does it have color and graphics that provide a welcome relief from a screen with nothing but print on it? How does the computer respond to wrong answers; is the response helpful? If they make a mistake in following directions, can students extricate themselves from the situation without starting over? Would students see the program as repetitious of classroom and textbook material or as a broadening application of material already learned? If the program is repetitious of classroom content but presents the material in a better way, the instructor may want to consider using the computer program to provide the lesson and using class time to expand on the subject in another creative way.

Software reviews often appear in nursing magazines, and this trend will probably continue to grow. Thus, some of the ground-work on evaluation of software will already be done for the educa-tor on the lookout for good programs. Locating software was once a problem, but it is becoming much easier with the increased interest in computer use for nursing. Textbook publishers who produce computer software advertise in many of the nursing maga-zines, and nurse-user groups, which are springing up around the country, can be helpful in providing information about software.

One note for staff development educators: relatively few hospi-tal education departments have microcomputers for teaching pur-poses. Because of the high costs involved, purchasing several com-puters and a lot of software may not be feasible. It might be possible, however, to purchase one computer and a few software programs, which could be justified on the basis of frequent use. The purchase of an overhead projector display palette can enable an instructor to project the computer screen onto a regular screen (by means of an overhead projector) for group instruction. Assuming that the programs purchased would be appropriate for use by small groups, this approach might be one way to incorporate CAI at relatively low cost. The display palette can be useful in schools of nursing as well, especially in demonstrating the use of a software package before the students use it individually.

Teaching strategies in the field of nursing should keep pace with the growth of the technologies in our society. Nursing facul-ties have to be familiar with educational and practice applications of the technologies and be open to learning and experimentation with them. Instructors need not be intimidated by the equipment but rather should learn how to use it and master it to enhance their teaching.

Research on Computer-Assisted Instruction

Several studies have been reported in which no differences were found in final exam scores between groups taught by CAI and those taught by traditional methods. In each of these studies, how-ever, the researchers reported that CAI groups learned the content in much less time (Bitzer & Boudreaux, 1969; Braun, 1980; Axeen, 1967 and Homeyer, 1970 cited in Jamison et al, 1974; Neil, 1985).

Hagerty, in 1970, also found no significant difference in performance of graduate students taught by computer versus those taught by lecture, but he did find that the computer instruction cost less than the conventional lecture method (cited in Jamison et al, 1974).

A slightly different outcome was obtained by Castelberry and Lagowski in 1970 (cited in Jamison et al, 1974). In their chemistry course, students who took advantage of the CAI modules scored significantly higher on the final examination.

Looking at transfer of learning as well as final exam results, Huckabay et al (1979) investigated the performance of nurse practitioner students taught the care of a hypertensive patient by CAI as opposed to a group taught by lecture/discussion. They found no significant difference on these outcomes.

Kirchoff and Holzemer (1979) studied the effectiveness of a PLATO program in teaching postoperative nursing care to 100 nursing students at the University of Illinois. No control group of students was used, but the researchers found that the students did learn the material by this method. They also found no correlation between the learning style of the students and the amount of learning through CAI.

Kulik, Kulik, and Cohen (1980) did a meta-analysis of 59 studies on CAI at the college level (including some of the research already cited). They were able to draw several conclusions. First, in 37 of 54 studies, students taught by CAI performed better on examinations than students taught by conventional instruction. In 13 cases, the superior performance of the CAI groups was statistically significant. Second, in 8 of 11 studies that compared student attitudes toward CAI and conventional classes, CAI was rated higher by students than was conventional instruction. Four of the 11 attitude studies showed a statistically significant difference in favor of CAI, and only 1 study did so in favor of conventional classes. Third, in the 8 studies devoted to comparing the amount of time spent in CAI and in conventional instruction, a substantial time savings was documented for CAI. On the average, conventional instruction consumed about 3.5 hours per week as compared to 2.25 hours per week for CAI.

In 1981 Larson (cited in Murphy, 1984) evaluated the use of a computer simulation of intravenous rate calculations and regulations and found that students learning by this method performed these tasks as well as students who learned in a nursing skills laboratory. Also, the CAI group completed the material in significantly shorter time and at less cost to the institution.

Day and Payne (1984) compared the performance of two groups of nursing students taught health assessment by CAI and by lecture. The two methods were found to be equally effective, but the majority of students had a negative attitude toward CAI. Indeed, 69% of the students preferred lectures over CAI, although 23% suggested using a combination of both methods. In a 1986 nursing study, however, Thiele reported that nursing students who had been taught drug calculations by means of a CAI package not only performed better than the lecture group but had very positive attitudes toward CAI.

Several conclusions can be drawn from the research evidence to date. Although there are some conflicting results, and not all of the studies were tightly controlled, it seems safe to say that CAI is at least as effective as traditional instruction and perhaps more effective in teaching certain subject matter at certain levels of Bloom's taxonomy. CAI also saves instructional time and, after the initial cost of hardware, may save money. Student attitudes toward CAI are generally favorable.

Computers have an undeniably important place in the education of today's nursing students. That does not mean that entire courses need to be taught in the form of CAI, but certainly many courses would be enhanced by its use. Further research needs to move beyond just testing the effectiveness of CAI compared to other methods of instruction, to find how CAI can be implemented and integrated to the best advantage. For example, is CAI more effective when used as an adjunct to classroom teaching or when it is used as a replacement for in-class instruction? Are CAI programs more effective when graphics are included? Do clinical simulations on computers enhance students' problem-solving abilities? How true to life are computerized clinical simulations, and can the learning transfer to the real world? The answers to these and other questions would help educators use this medium more wisely.

References

Bitzer MD, Boudreaux MC: Using a computer to teach nursing. *Nurs Forum* 1969; 8:234–254.

Braun L: Computers in learning environments: an imperative for the 1980s. *Byte* 1980; 5:101–114.

Brose CH: Computer technology in nursing: revolution or renaissance? *Nurs Health Care* 1984; 5:531–534.

Collart ME: Computer-assisted instruction and the teaching-learning process. *Nurs Outlook* 1973; 21:527–532.

Day R, Payne L: Comparison of lecture presentation versus computer-managed instruction. *Computers in Nurs* 1984; 6:236–240.

Edmunds L: Computerized information systems. In Atkinson LD, Murray ME, *Fundamentals of Nursing*. Macmillan, 1985.

Huckabay LMD et al: Cognitive, affective, and transfer of learning consequences of computer-assisted instruction. *Nurs Res* 1979; 28:228–233.

Jamison D, Suppes P, Wells S: The effectiveness of alternative instructional media: a survey. *Rev Educ Res* (Winter) 1974; 44:1–67.

Jenkins TM, Dankert EJ: Results of a three-month PLATO trial in terms of utilization and student attitudes. *Educ Tech* (March) 1981; 21:44–47.

Kirchoff KT, Holzemer WL: Student learning and a computer-assisted instructional program. *J Nurs Educ* (March) 1979; 18:22–30.

Kulik JA, Kulik CC, Cohen PA: Effectiveness of computer-based college teaching: a meta-analysis of findings. *Rev Educ Res* 1980; 50:525–544.

Lorenz M, Moose A: Writing instructional software. *MICRO* 1983; 64:44–49.

Mahr DR, Kadner KD: Computer-aided instruction: overview and relevance to nursing education. *J Nurs Educ* 1984; 23:366–368.

Murphy MA: Computer-based education in nursing. *Computers in Nurs* 1984; 2:218–223.

Neil RM: Effects of computer-assisted instruction on nursing student learning and attitude. *J Nurs Educ* 1985; 24:72–75.

Reynolds AJ: Using microcomputers in situational testing. *Nurse Educator* (Summer) 1984; 9:39–42.

Smith JM: Courseware evaluation. *Computers in Nurs* 1985; 3:117–121.

Thiele J: The development of computer-assisted instruction for drug dosage calculations. *Computers in Nurs* 1986; 4:114–118.

Thiele JE, Baldwin JH: A simulated practice environment. *Computers in Nurs* 1985; 3:113–116.

Van Dongen CJ, Van Dongen WO: Using microcomputers to teach psychopharmacology. *J Nurs Educ* 1984; 23:259–260.

Ziemer MM: Issues of computer literacy in nursing education. *Nurs Health Care* 1984; 5:537–542.

Additional References

Chapter 1   The Good Teacher

Dawson N: Hours of contact and their relationship to students' evaluations of teaching effectiveness. *J Nurs Educ* 1986; 25:236-239.

Fogarty JL, Wang MC, Creek R: A descriptive study of experienced and novice teachers' interactive instructional thoughts and actions. *J Educ Res* 1983; 77:22-32.

Granrose JT: Conscious teaching: helping graduate assistants develop teaching styles. Pages 21-30 in: *Improving Teaching Styles*. Eble KE (editor). Jossey-Bass, 1980.

Griffith JW, Bakanauskas AJ: Student-instructor relationships in nursing education. *J Nurs Educ* 1983; 22:104–107.

Hammer RM, Tufts MA: Nursing's self-image—nursing education's responsibility. *J Nurs Educ* 1985; 24:280–283.

Hassenplug LW: The good teacher. *Nurs Outlook* 1965; 13:24–27.

Layton MM: How instructors' attitudes affect students. *Nurs Outlook* 1969; 17:27–29.

McKeachie WJ, Lin Y, Mann W: Student ratings of teacher effectiveness: validity studies. *Amer Educ Res Journal* 1971; 8:435–445.

McKeithan Ripley D: Invitational teaching behaviors in the associate degree clinical setting. *J Nurs Educ* 1986; 25:240–246.

Mims FH: Students evaluate faculty. *Nurs Outlook* 1970; 18:53–55.

Pugh EJ; Dynamics of teaching-learning interaction. *Nurs Forum* 1976; 15:49–58.

Van Ort SR: Developing a system for documenting teaching effectiveness. *J Nurs Educ* 1983; 22:324–328.

Zimmerman L, Waltman N: Effective clinical behaviors of faculty: a review of the literature. *Nurse Educator* (Jan/Feb) 1986; 11:31–34.

Zimmerman L, Westfall J: The development and validation of a scale measuring effective clinical teaching behaviors. *J Nurs Educ* 1988; 27:274–277.

Chapter 2   The Learning Process

Bevis ED: *Curriculum Building in Nursing.* Mosby, 1973.
Brodie B: Reexamination of reinforcement in the learning process. *J Nurs Educ* (April) 1969; 8:27–30.
Brown AL et al: Learning, remembering, and understanding. Chapter 2 in: *Handbook of Child Psychology,* 4th ed. Vol 3: Cognitive Development. Mussen PH (editor). Wiley, 1983.
Conklin KR: Foundations of education for students and teachers of nursing. *J Nurs Educ* (Aug) 1974; 13:16–22.
Eble KE: *The Craft of Teaching.* Jossey-Bass, 1976.
Hyman RT: *Ways of Teaching.* Lippincott, 1974.
McKeachie WJ: *Teaching Tips: A Guidebook for the Beginning College Teacher.* Heath, 1969.
Schweer JE: *Creative Teaching in Clinical Nursing.* Mosby, 1968.
Shetland ML: Teaching and learning in nursing. *Am J Nurs* 1965; 65:112–116.
Strike KA: The logic of learning by discovery. *Rev Educ Res* 1975; 45:461–483.
Weimer RC: An analysis of discovery. *Educ Tech* 1975; 15:45–48.

Chapter 3   Planning and Conducting Classes

Bevis EO: *Curriculum Building in Nursing.* Mosby, 1978.
Cranston CM, McCort B: A learner analysis experiment: cognitive style versus learning style in undergraduate nursing education. *J Nurs Educ* 1985; 24:136–138.
DeCecco JP: *The Psychology of Learning and Instruction.* Prentice-Hall, 1968.
deTornyay R: Instructional technology and nursing education. *J Nurs Educ* (April) 1970; 9:3–8,34.
Frank BM: Cognitive styles and teacher education: field dependence and areas of specialization among teacher education majors. *J Educ Res* (Sept/Oct) 1986; 80:19–22.
Heye ML et al: A textbook selection process. *Nurse Educator* (Jan/Feb) 1987; 12:14–18.
Phillips C, Harman E: Criteria for selecting textbooks. *Nurse Educator* (March/April) 1986; 11:31–34.

Chapter 4   Lecture, Discussion, Questioning

Andre T: Does answering higher-level questions while reading facilitate productive learning? *Rev Educ Res* 1979; 49:280–318.
Crow ML: Teaching as an interactive process. Pages 41–55 in: *Improving Teaching Styles.* Eble KE (editor). Jossey-Bass, 1980.

Egan K: How to ask questions that promote high-level thinking. *Peabody J Educ* 1975; 52:228–234.

Hayter J: How good is the lecture as a teaching method? *Nurs Outlook* 1979; 27:274–277.

Hunkins FP: Using questions to foster pupils' thinking. *Education* 1966; 87:83–87.

Thompson R: Legitimate lecturing. *Improving College and University Teaching* 1974; 22:163–164.

Vavoulis A: Lecture vs. discussion. *Improving College and University Teaching* 1964; 12:185–189.

Chapter 5   Seminar, Brainstorming, Debate

Archbold PA, Hoeffer B: Reframing the issue: a debate on third-party reimbursement. *Nurs Outlook* 1981; 29:423–425.

Baldonado A: Creative teaching-learning strategies. *J Contin Educ Nurs* (May/June) 1979; 10:11–16.

Cooper SS: Methods of teaching revisited: brainstorming. *J Contin Educ Nurs* (Nov/Dec) 1978; 9:16–18.

Cooper SS: Methods of teaching revisited: formal discussion: the debate. *J Contin Educ Nurs* (July/Aug) 1979; 10:58,71.

Gesse T, Dempsey P: Debate as a teaching-learning strategy. *Nurs Outlook* 1981; 29:421–423.

Pender NJ: The debate as a teaching and learning tool. *Nurs Outlook* 1967; 15:42–43.

Schweer JE: *Creative Teaching in Clinical Nursing.* Mosby, 1968.

Chapter 6   Individualized Learning

Armstrong ML, Toebe DM, Watson MR: Strengthening the instructional role in self-directed learning activities. *J Contin Educ Nurs* (May/June) 1985; 16:75–79.

Beyers M, Dieklemann N, Thompson M: Developing a modular curriculum. *Nurs Outlook* 1972; 20:643–647.

Blatchley ME, Herzog PM, Russell JD: The media center: it's great, but . . . *J Nurs Educ* (Jan) 1978; 17:24–28.

Blatchley ME, Herzog PM, Russell JD: Effects of self-study on achievement in a medical-nursing course. *Nurs Outlook* 1978; 26:444–447.

Buterbaugh JG, Fuller RG: Personalized system of instruction (PSI): an alternative. *Audiovisual Instruction* (March) 1975; 20:62–65.

Cowart ME, Burge JM: Evaluation by jury. *Nurs Outlook* 1979; 27:329–333.

deTornyay R, Thompson MA: *Strategies for Teaching Nursing,* 3d ed. Wiley, 1987.

Ferrell B: Attitudes toward learning styles and self-direction of ADN students. *J Nurs Educ* (Feb) 1978; 17:19–22.

Langford T: Self-directed learning. *Nurs Outlook* 1972; 20:648–651.

Magidson EM: Is your module good? How do you know? *Audiovisual Instruction* (Oct) 1976; 21:43–44.

Mast ME, VanAlta MJ: Applying adult learning principles in instructional module design. *Nurse Educator* (Jan/Feb) 1986; 11:35–39.

O'Connor ME, Jones D: An innovative teaching strategy for nursing education. *J Nurs Educ* (Nov) 1975; 14:9–15.

Osborn WP, Thompson MA: Variables associated with student mastery of learning modules. *Communicating Nurs Res* 1976; 9:167–179.

Perry SE: Teaching strategy and learner performance. *J Nurs Educ* (Jan) 1979; 18:25–27.

Spickerman S, Lee BT, Eason FR: Use of learning modules to teach nursing leadership concepts. *J Nurs Educ* 1988; 27:78–82.

Chapter 7   Learning Through Simulation

Anderson LF: *A Comparison of Simulation, Case Studies, and Problem Papers in Teaching Decision Making.* ERIC Document #001231, 1964.

Armistead C: How useful are case studies? *Training and Development J* 1984; 38:75–77.

Boocock SS, Schild EO: *Simulation Games in Learning.* Sage, 1968.

Boreham NC: The use of case histories to assess nurses' ability to solve clinical problems. *J Adv Nurs* 1977; 2:57–66.

Cherryholmes C: Developments in simulation of international relations in high school teaching. *Phi Delta Kappan* 1965; 46:227–231.

Cooper SS: Methods of teaching revisited: games and simulation. *J Contin Educ Nurs* (Sept/Oct) 1979; 10:14,47–48.

Cooper SS: Methods of teaching revisited: role playing. *J Contin Educ Nurs* (Jan/Feb) 1980; 11:36,57–58.

Cooper SS: Methods of teaching revisited: case method. *J Contin Educ Nurs* (Sept/Oct) 1981; 12:32–36.

Crancer J, Maury-Hess S: Games: an alternative to pedagogical instruction. *J Nurs Educ* (March) 1980; 19:45-52.

Curtis J, Rothert M: An instructional simulation system offering practice in assessment of patient needs. *J Nurs Educ* (Jan) 1972; 11:23–28.

Davidhizar RE: Use of simulation games in teaching psychiatric nursing. *J Nurs Educ* (May) 1977; 16:9–12.

Dearth S, McKenzie L: Synoptics: a simulation game for health professional students. *J Contin Educ Nurs* (July/Aug) 1975; 6:28–31.

Dunathan AT: What is a game? *Audiovisual Instruction* (May) 1978; 23:14–15.

Hoban JD: Successful simulations for health education. *Audiovisual Instruction* (Dec) 1978; 23:20–22.

Huston C, Marquis B: Use of management and ethical case studies to improve decision-making skills in senior nursing students. *J Nurs Educ* 1987; 26:210–212.

Johnson J, Purvis J: Case studies: an alternative learning/teaching method in nursing. *J Nurs Educ* 1987; 26:118–120.

McDonald GF: The simulated clinical laboratory. *Nurs Outlook* 1987; 35:290–292.

McKeachie WJ: *Teaching Tips: A Guidebook for the Beginning College Teacher.* DC Heath, 1969.

Mitchell JJ: The use of case studies in bioethics courses. *J Nurs Educ* (Nov) 1981; 20:31–36.

O'Connell AL, Bates B: The case method in nurse practitioner education. *Nurs Outlook* 1976; 24:243–246.

Pearson BD: Simulation techniques for nursing education. *Internat Nurs Rev* 1975; 22:144–146.

Perry LC: The use of simulation with students having a community health nursing experience. *J Nurs Educ* (April) 1973; 12:20–25.

Plasterer HH, Mills N: Teach management theory—through fun and games. *J Nurs Educ* 1983; 22:80–83.

Rothkopf C, Tessier D: How to design simulation games. *Audiovisual Instruction* 1978; 23:28–30.

Spannaus TW: What is a simulation? *Audiovisual Instruction* 1978; 23:16–17.

Swendsen Boss LA: Teaching for clinical competence. *Nurse Educator* (July/ Aug) 1985; 10:8–12.

Tarcinale MA: The case study as a vicarious learning technique. *J Nurs Educ* 1987; 26:340–341.

Walts NS: Games and simulations. *Nurs Management* 1982; 13:28–29.

Whitis G: Simulation in teaching clinical nursing. *J Nurs Educ* 1985; 24:161–163.

Wynn R: Simulation: terrible reality in the preparation of school administrators. *Phi Delta Kappan* 1964; 46:170–173.

Chapter 8   Psychomotor Skills

Clark LV: Effect of mental practice on the development of a certain motor skill. *Res Quarterly* 1960; 31:560–569.

Cook JW, Hill PM: The impact of successful laboratory system on the teaching of nursing skills. *J Nurs Educ* 1985; 24:344–346.

Cowan D, Wiens V: Mock hospital: a preclinical laboratory experience. *Nurse Educator* (Sept/Oct) 1986; 11:30–32.

Eaton SL: *The Influence of Mental Imagery on the Performance of a Complex Psychomotor Nursing Skill Using Two Learning Approaches.* (Doctoral dissertation.) University of San Francisco, 1984.

Hanson R: Motor skill acquisition in nursing. *Nursing Papers* 1977; 9:68–75.

Hegstad LN, Zsohar H: A study of the cost-effectiveness of providing psychomotor practice in teaching intravenous infusion techniques. *J Nurs Educ* 1986; 25:10–14.

Kieffer JS: Selecting technical skills to teach for competency. *J Nurs Educ* 1984; 23:196–203.

Mast DE: Effects of imagery. *Image* 1986; 18:118–120.

Megel ME, Wilken MK, Volcek MK: Nursing students' performance: administering injections in laboratory and clinical area. *J Nurs Educ* 1987; 26:288–293.

Patel AS, Grant DA: Decrement and recovery effects in a perceptual-motor learning task as a function of effort, distribution of practice, and sex of subject. *J General Psych* 1964; 71:217–231.

Robb MD: *The Dynamics of Motor-Skill Acquisition.* Prentice-Hall, 1972.

Schweer JE: *Creative Teaching in Clinical Nursing.* Mosby, 1968.

Singer RN: *Readings in Motor Learning.* Lea & Febiger, 1972.

Chapter 9   Clinical Laboratory Teaching

Bevil CW, Gross LL: Assessing the adequacy of clinical learning settings. *Nurs Outlook* 1981; 29:658–661.

Blomquist KB: Evaluation of students: intuition is important. *Nurse Educator* (Nov/Dec) 1985; 10:8–11.

delBueno DJ: Performance evaluation: when all is said and done, more is said than done. *J Nurs Admin* (Dec) 1977; 7:21–23.

Hatrock B: Multiple student assignments. *Nurs Outlook* (Nov) 1969; 17:40–42.

Hawkins JW: *Clinical Experiences in Collegiate Nursing Education.* Springer, 1981.

Holzemer WL (editor): *Review of Research in Nursing Education.* SLACK, 1983.

Jenkins HM: Improving clinical decision making in nursing. *J Nurs Educ* 1985; 24:242–243.

Joachim G, Karampelas A: Head nurse and clinical instructor. *Canad Nurse* (Feb) 1982; 78:26–29.

Lewis EP: Quantifying the unquantifiable. *Nurs Outlook* 1976; 24:147.

Little D, Carnevali D: Complexities of teaching in the clinical laboratory. *J Nurs Educ* (Jan) 1972; 11:15–22.

Litwack L: A system for evaluation. *Nurs Outlook* 1976; 24:45–48.

McCabe BW: The improvement of instruction in the clinical area: a challenge waiting to be met. *J Nurs Educ* 1985; 24:255–257.

Meleca CB et al: Clinical instruction in nursing: a national survey. *J Nurs Educ* (Oct)1981; 20:32–40.

Novak S: An effective clinical evaluation tool. *J Nurs Educ* 1988; 27:83–84.

Olson EM: Baccalaureate students' perceptions of factors assisting knowledge application in the clinical laboratory. *J Nurs Educ* 1983; 22:18–21.

Smith DW: *Perspectives on Clinical Teaching,* 2d ed. Springer, 1977.

Tanner CA, Lindeman CA: Research in nursing education: assumptions and priorities. *J Nurs Educ* 1987; 26:57–59.

Turkoski B: Reducing stress in nursing students' clinical learning experience. *J Nurs Educ* 1987; 26:335–337.

Wang AM, Blumberg P: A study on interaction techniques of nursing faculty in the clinical area. *J Nurs Educ* 1983; 22:144–151.

Woolley AS: The long and tortured history of clinical evaluation. *Nurs Outlook* 1977; 25:308–315.

Chapter 10   Audiovisual Technology in the Classroom

Bauman K, Kunka AK: Overhead transparencies: the overlooked medium. *Nurse Educator* (July/Aug) 1979; 4:21–25.

Blatchley ME, Herzog PM, Russell JD: The media center: it's great, but . . . . *J Nurs Educ* (Jan) 1978; 17:24–33.

Brown JW, Lewis RB, Harcleroad FF: *AV Instruction: Media and Methods.* McGraw-Hill, 1969.

Browning EM, Campbell ME: Evaluating students' communication skills: tape recording. *Nurse Educator* (Jan/Feb) 1987; 12:28–29.

Carlson DS: Self-produced programs as an alternative to purchasing audiovisual materials. *J Contin Educ Nurs* 1988; 19:76–77.

Carver J: Effective use of the overhead projector. *Canad Nurse* (July/Aug) 1982; 78:54.

Cooper S: Methods of teaching revisited: the overhead projector. *J Contin Educ Nurs* (May/June) 1980; 11:56,71–72.

Cooper S: Methods of teaching revisited: slides and slide-sound presentations. *J Contin Educ Nurs* (Sept/Oct) 1980; 11:52–55.

Cooper S: Methods of teaching revisited: films and videotapes. *J Contin Educ Nurs* (Jan/Feb) 1981; 12:34–37.

Dalgarno J: A guide to the overhead projector–1. *Nurs Times* 1980; 76:1482–1483.

Dalgarno J: Guide to the overhead projector–2. *Nurs Times* 1980; 76:1669–1670.

Dalgarno J: Achieving good projection. *Nurs Times* 1980; 76:1834–1835.

Dalgarno J: Producing your own teaching material. *Nurs Times* 1980; 76:2068–2070.

Dalgarno J: Producing a programme on videotape and taking care of the equipment. *Nurs Times* 1980; 76:2250–2251.

Dalgarno J: It won't work. *Nurs Times* 1981; 77:120–121.

deTornyay R, Thompson MA: *Strategies for Teaching Nursing,* 3d ed. Wiley, 1987.

Donaldson ML: Instructional media as a teaching strategy. *Nurse Educator* (July/Aug) 1979; 4:18–20.

Duane NF: An audiovisual overview. *Nurse Educator* (July/Aug) 1979; 4:7–10.

Forsyth DN: Assisting in the development of a slidetape: a learning experience. *J Nurs Educ* (April) 1980; 19:42–45.

Gustafson MB, Corcoran SA: *TDR Teachers' Desk Reference.* Medical Economics, 1978.

Hofland SL: Transparency design for effective oral presentations. *J Contin Educ Nurs* 1987; 18:83–88.

Jamison D, Suppes P, Wells S: The effectiveness of alternative instructional media: a survey. *Rev Educ Res* (Winter) 1974; 44:1–67.

Kerpelman LC: Films in nursing education. *Nurs Outlook* 1975; 23:35–37.

Koch HB: Television in nursing education. *J Nurs Educ* (April) 1968; 7:37–43.

Kodak Motion Picture and Audiovisual Markets Division: *Effective Lecture Slides.* Kodak Publication No. s–22. Eastman Kodak, 1982.

Moser DH, Kondracki MR: Comparison of attitudes and cognitive achievement of nursing students in three instructional strategies. *J Nurs Educ* (Jan) 1977; 16:14–28.

Myers LB, Greenwood SE: Use of traditional and autotutorial instruction in fundamentals of nursing courses. *J Nurs Educ* (March) 1978; 17:7–13.

Oermann MH: Analyzing and selecting audiovisual materials. *Nurse Educator* (Winter) 1984; 9:24–27.

Pittman PR: Videotaping : a technique for teaching basic communication skills. *Nurse Educator* (Nov/Dec) 1977; 2:16–17.

Reed SD: The overhead projector and transparencies. *J Nurs Educ* (April) 1968; 7:9–14.

Reiser RA, Gagne RM: Characteristics of media selection models. *Rev Educ Res* 1982; 52:499–512.

Schmalenberg C: Making and using slides. *Nurse Educator* (July/Aug) 1979; 4:12–15.

Shaffer MK, Pfeiffer IL: Videotape as a method for staff development of nurses. *J Contin Educ Nurs* (Nov/Dec) 1978; 9:19–24.

Shaffer SM, Indorato KL, Deneselya JA: *Teaching in Schools of Nursing.* Mosby, 1972.

Sparks SM, Mitchell GE: The national medical audiovisual center. *J Nurs Educ* (Jan) 1978; 17:29–34.

Stewart PH: Utilizing slides in the learning experience. *Nurse Educator* (July/Aug) 1981; 6:9–11.

Stuck DL, Manatt RP: A comparison of audio-tutorial and lecture methods of teaching. *J Educ Res* 1970; 63:414–418.

Valentine NM, Saito Y: Videotaping: a viable teaching strategy in nursing education. *Nurse Educator* (July/Aug) 1980; 5:8–17.

Van Hoozer H, Brink PJ, Opplinger R: The effects of overhead transparency design on retention, recall, and application of data analysis content. *J Nurs Educ* 1989; 28:181–187.

Chapter 11   Computer Technology

Ahijevych K, Boyle KK, Burger K: Microcomputers enhance student health fairs. *J Nurs Educ* 1985; 24:16–20.

Billings DM: Evaluating computer-assisted instruction. *Nurs Outlook* 1984; 32:50–53.

Bork A: Computers in the classroom. Chapter 7 in: *On College Teaching*. Milton O and Associates. Jossey-Bass, 1978.

Day R, Payne L: Computer-managed instruction: an alternative teaching strategy. *J Nurs Educ* 1987; 26:30–36.

Donabedian D: Computer-taught epidemiology. *Nurs Outlook* 1976; 24:749–751.

Edwards J et al: How effective is CAI? A review of the research. *Educ Leadership* 1975; 33:147–153.

Felton BB: Planning and implementing computer learning in a department of nursing. *Nurs Health Care* 1984; 5:549–553.

Gaston S: Knowledge, retention, and attitude effects of computer-assisted instruction. *J Nurs Educ* 1988; 27:30–34.

Gerhold G: Teaching with a microcomputer. *Byte* 1978; 3:124–126.

Goodwin JO, Edwards BS: Developing a computer program to assist the nursing process: phase 1—from systems analysis to an expandable program. *Nurs Res* 1975; 24:299–305.

Grobe SJ: Computer-assisted instruction. *Computers in Nurs* 1984; 2:92–97.

Hamby CS: A study of the effects of computer-assisted instruction on the attitude and achievement of vocational nursing students. *Computers in Nurs* 1986; 4:109–113.

Hassett MR: Computers and nursing education in the 1980s. *Nurs Outlook*, 1984; 32:34–36.

Hebda T: A profile of the use of computer-assisted instruction within baccalaureate nursing education. *Computers in Nurs* 1988; 6:22–29.

Heller BR et al: Computer applications in nursing. *Computers in Nurs* 1985; 3:14–22.

Holzemer WL et al: Development of a computer resources facility. *Nurs Health Care* 1984; 5:545–547.

Howard EP: Use of a computer simulation for the continuing education of registered nurses. *Computers in Nurs* 1987; 5:208–213.

Kamp M, Burnside IM: Computer-assisted learning in graduate psychiatric nursing. *J Nurs Educ* (Nov) 1974; 13:18–25.

Kellogg B, Garcia S: Introducing nursing students to computers. *Computers in Nurs* 1985; 3:128–132.

McColgan JJ: A computer program to test drug dosage calculation abilities. *Nurs Health Care* 1984; 5:555–558.

Meadows LS: Nursing education in crisis: a computer alternative. *J Nurs Educ* (May) 1977; 16:13–21.

Mirin S: The computer's place in nursing education. *Nurs Health Care* 1981; 2:500–506.

Newman MA: Experiencing the research process via computer simulation. *Image* 1978; 10:5–9.

Ronald JS: Computers and undergraduate nursing education: a report on an experimental introductory course. *J Nurs Educ* (Nov) 1979; 18:4–9.

Ryan SA: An expert system for nursing practice. *Computers in Nurs* 1985; 3:77–84.

Schleutermann JA, Holzemer WL, Farrand LL: An evaluation of paper-and-pencil and computer-assisted simulations. *J Nurs Educ* 1983; 22:315–323.

Sumida SW: A computerized test for clinical decision making. *Nurs Outlook* 1972; 20:458-461.

Timpke J, Janney CP: Teaching drug dosages by computer. *Nurs Outlook* 1981; 29:376–377.

Van Dongen CJ: Creating relevant computer-assisted instruction. *Nurse Educator* (Jan/Feb) 1985; 10:21–25.

Woodbury PA, Ayers JL: Interpersonal skill development: a computer-assisted approach. *Nurse Educator* (Autumn) 1984; 9:30–36.

Index